Menopause

A report by the
Special Advisory Committee on
Reproductive Physiology
to the Drugs Directorate
Health Protection Branch
Health Canada

The views expressed in this publication are those
of the Special Advisory Committee on
Reproductive Physiology and do not necessarily
reflect those of Health Canada.

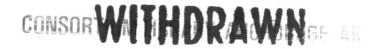

Our mission is to help the people of Canada
maintain and improve their health.

Health Canada

Published by authority of the Minister of
National Health and Welfare

©Minister of Supply and Services Canada 1995
Cat. H42-2/67-1995E
ISBN 0-660-15911-2

Également disponible en français sous le titre
La ménopause

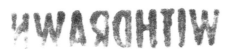

Special Advisory Committee on Reproductive Physiology

Chairperson
Dr. Robert F. Casper, Toronto, Ontario

Vice Chairperson
Dr. Mariette Morin-Gonthier, Montreal, Quebec

Dr. Marilynne Bell, Halifax, Nova Scotia
Dr. Cedric J. Carter, Vancouver, British Columbia
Dr. Lindsay Edouard, Saskatoon, Saskatchewan
Dr. Yves Lefebvre, Montreal, Quebec
Dr. André Lemay, Quebec, Quebec
Dr. Nadia Z. Mikhael, Ottawa, Ontario
Dr. T.M. Roulston, Winnipeg, Manitoba (deceased, June 1994)
Dr. A. Albert Yuzpe, London, Ontario

Executive Secretary
Dr. André-Marie Leroux, Health Protection Branch

Acknowledgements

The assistance of the following former members of the Special Advisory Committee on Reproductive Physiology is gratefully acknowledged: Dr. Janice M. Boxall, Dr. Mary Ellen Kirk, Dr. Betty J. Poland (deceased), Dr. Earl R. Plunkett, and Dr. Jack H. Walters (former Chairperson).

The participation of the following consultants is much appreciated: Dr. John D. Gay, Dr. Anthony B. Miller, Dr. Greg O'Connell (on behalf of The Society of Gynecologic Oncologists of Canada), Dr. Henri Bélanger, Dr. Carl E. Boyd (former Executive Secretary of the Committee), and Dr. Peter Grosser (editorial advisor), Terry Chernis (librarian), and Adele Boulais-Thomas (secretary). A review of this document by the Society of Obstetricians and Gynecologists of Canada was very helpful.

Foreword

The objective of this publication is to provide physicians and other health care givers with important information on drugs that could be used as part of the comprehensive care of women entering into or in menopause. This publication is the result of the enthusiasm and sustained teamwork of the medical experts in reproductive physiology appointed as consultants to the Bureau of Human Prescription Drugs. It represents their opinions on the drugs that could be used when a physician has concluded that such treatment is warranted.

It is not the intention of the Bureau to advocate or refute the use of drugs in the management of the symptoms of menopause. That decision should be taken only after a thorough physical examination and subsequent discussion between the woman and her physician of the benefits and risks associated with the use of these medications and of other possible non-pharmaceutical interventions.

I wish to thank the members of the Special Advisory Committee on Reproductive Physiology and all the other contributors for their dedication to seeing this project through to completion.

Claire A. Franklin, Ph.D.
Director,
Bureau of Human Prescription Drugs

Table of Contents

1. Introduction

During the last two decades, the approach to the management of the menopausal and postmenopausal woman has undergone significant changes. The use of long-term hormone replacement therapy (HRT) has become increasingly popular, as attention has focused on delaying the progression of osteoporosis and preventing cardiovascular disease.

Public awareness of menopause has been increased lately by lay publications such as *The Silent Passage* by Gail Sheehy.[1] Similarly, the lay press has educated the public, though not always accurately, and has raised the patient's expectations of therapy. Reports on side effects and complications of long-term therapy have received wide circulation, and have not always reflected the benefits of replacement therapy.

The range of symptoms that perimenopausal women may voice, and concerns about hormonal therapy, present the doctor/patient relationship with considerable difficulty in decisions regarding treatment. This publication has been produced to review briefly some of the latest medical opinions and knowledge, in the hope that it may help to clarify the situation.

Appropriate counselling forms an important part of any therapy. Medication, whether short-term or long-term, remains to be decided by the individual practitioner and the patient, based upon full knowledge of the benefits and risks.

Menopause

Menopause is commonly defined as the last occurrence of physiological uterine bleeding (menstruation). It should, however, be considered as one event in the process of change from reproductive to non-reproductive life, the climacteric. The perimenopause includes the first few years of the climacteric and the first year after menopause. The average age of onset of menopause is around 50 years, and appears to be unrelated to race, socioeconomic status, physical characteristics, or the date of the last pregnancy. Spontaneous cessation of menstruation before the age of 45 years is known as premature menopause. Total removal of ovarian function by surgery or radiotherapy during the reproductive years results in artificial menopause, in contrast to natural menopause. Since average life expectancy for women in Canada is now approximately 80 years, the number of adult years spent postmenopausally is almost equal to the number of years spent in the reproductive period.

Cause

While the exact mechanism of the normal menopause is not completely known, the primary cause lies in the ovary and is related to the depletion of the primordial follicles by atresia and their loss of sensitivity to stimuli from the pituitary gonadotropins. In the perimenopausal period, ovulatory cycles become sporadic and the subsequent anovulatory cycles result in irregular and sometimes heavy bleeding. As follicle numbers and sensitivity are further reduced, despite rising levels of serum follicle stimulating hormone (FSH) and luteinizing hormone (LH), estrogen levels fall and irregular periods with longer intermenstrual intervals give way to permanent amenorrhea with an atrophic endometrium. Occasionally, the onset of menopause abruptly follows regular menstruation, so that the premenopausal pattern is absent.

A diagnosis of menopause can be made if there is one year of amenorrhea in late reproductive life. This can be substantiated on the basis of increased serum FSH levels over 40 IU/L.

Throughout the climacteric and after menopause, as changes affect the genital and other systems, it should be remembered that the aging process and its effect on the psyche and soma continue. Further, the climacteric often coincides with significant changes within the woman's family and workplace and her socioeconomic status, all of which may affect the presenting features when the patient seeks help from the physician.

Up to 85% of women will experience symptoms related to estrogen deficiency, though the number who seek help is considerably less. Acceptance of menopausal and postmenopausal symptoms varies among cultures.

Clinical Manifestations

The main groups of symptoms which affect women are due largely to estrogen deprivation.

Hot flushes

Seventy-five to 85% of postmenopausal women will complain of hot flushes or flashes. These are experienced early in menopause and persist for some years. Fifty percent may have occasional flushes five and more years later. Some patients may experience flushes in the perimenopausal period prior to the onset of amenorrhea.

Episodic and lasting less than five minutes, the hot flush usually involves the chest, neck, and face, with a feeling of warmth which rapidly spreads to become generalized. Flushes are sometimes accompanied by palpitations or dizziness and by distressing and often profuse sweats, more commonly experienced at night. Sleep is often disturbed so that fatigue, lethargy, lack of concentration, and occasional depression are complaints.

Genitourinary changes and symptoms

Estrogen receptors are present in the vagina, vulva, urethra, bladder trigone, and in the vascular and neuronal supply to these areas. Estrogen deprivation results in significant changes such as vaginal dryness and burning, dyspareunia, discharge, and reduced blood flow to the vagina which may interfere with sexual function.

The uterus decreases in size and prolapse is more common after menopause. In part this may be due to estrogen deprivation with loss of pelvic supports and of elasticity. Hormone replacement therapy (HRT) prior to and following vaginal reparative surgery in the postmenopausal patient results in healthier vaginal tissues which enhance postoperative healing.

Changes in the urinary tract result in dysuria, urgency, frequency, and nocturia. Stress incontinence may become significant.

Osteoporosis

Osteoporosis is an abnormal rarefaction of bone resulting from a negative balance between deposition and resorption and leading to fractures. There are many causes for osteoporosis but this publication will refer only to the postmenopausal condition.

By age 50, both men and women have begun a generalized bone loss, but men have a greater bone mineral content which offers protection at least into the seventies or eighties. In women, bone loss following menopause or following bilateral oophorectomy at an earlier age may be as much as 4% per year for the first six years.

Osteoporosis is, therefore, not a complaint at the natural menopause. The insidious nature of the condition declares itself in skeletal fractures of the limbs and vertebral column, with increasing frequency after the age of 60. The mechanisms by which estrogen deprivation affect bone loss will be discussed in the section on Bone and Mineral Metabolism (Chapter 4).

Patients who fall into high-risk groups for development of severe osteoporosis include those with early loss of ovarian function due to surgery, radiation, or genetic abnormalities. Thin, white patients with fine bone structure, poor bone mass, and those with a family history of severe osteoporosis, also should be considered at high risk.

It should be noted that HRT in all postmenopausal patients cannot cure or prevent osteoporosis. It can only slow the process down as the condition progresses with age. Other measures are important adjuncts to estrogen replacement. A well-balanced diet with adequate calcium intake, weight-bearing exercise, and moderation in the use of caffeine and alcohol should be prescribed. Smoking should be discouraged.

Cardiovascular disease

It has been noted that males under age 55 have eight times the chance of developing coronary artery disease than females. However, after menopause, the rate of cardiovascular disease in women quickly increases and begins to approach the level seen in men. Atherosclerosis and vascular instability, leading to heart attacks and strokes, is the major cause of mortality and morbidity in postmenopausal women, far outweighing the risk of death from cancer and osteoporotic fractures combined. Estrogen replacement provides protection against atherosclerosis and cardiovascular disease and may reduce mortality in postmenopausal women by 50%. Prevention of cardiovascular disease is, therefore, one of the major factors to consider in therapy of menopause.

Endometrial cancer

One potential risk of estrogen therapy is the development of endometrial cancer, which may be increased three to five times. These cancers are low grade and treatment yields a 95% five-year survival. There is good evidence that the combination of estrogen with progestin protects the patient against endometrial cancer.

Breast cancer

Sufficient data exist at present to suggest there is an increased risk of breast cancer with long-term HRT. However, adequate information is not available to assess differences among the various types, dosages and schedules of administration of HRT. The magnitude of any increased risk is such that it is unlikely to outweigh the benefits of HRT. The data presented in these epidemiological studies do not warrant a change in the current prescribing practice of HRT at this time, but the need for further investigation and ongoing surveillance must be emphasized.

Summary

With this background in mind, the rest of this document will examine menopause and its management in more detail. Our intention in producing this report is to provide information and suggestions for the physician dealing with menopausal women. It is not our intention to produce guidelines or criteria with any medicolegal ramifications. Each physician must decide upon individualization of therapy according to the needs and wishes of the patient and in light of new information or products.

Reference

1.   Sheehy G., "*The Silent Passage: Menopause*," Random House of Canada Ltd., Toronto, 1992.

2.   Endocrinology of Menopause

Menopause is associated with events occurring over a long period of time before cessation of menses, and that should be included in the same phenomenon. Several years before menopause, there is an increase in the circulating levels of serum follicle stimulating hormone (FSH) and a decrease in the level of estradiol and progesterone.[1] FSH is particularly elevated during the early follicular phase; though the serum FSH level falls along with follicular maturation and estradiol secretion, it stays higher than in younger women, even in late luteal phase, while luteinizing hormone (LH) concentration remains in a normal range.

All of these changes frequently occur when ovulation is still present. The ovary gradually becomes less responsive to gonadotropins several years before menses cease, and this may be a triggering event in the initiation of menopause.[2] The small number of residual follicles left is probably the least sensitive to gonadal stimulation, and less likely to achieve complete maturation. With advancing age, the number of follicles diminishes, and the resistance to stimulation increases. Reduced ovarian follicular activity results in decreased production of estradiol and of inhibin by the ovary, which removes the negative feedback inhibition of gonadotropins, especially FSH production from the anterior pituitary.

As a result, serum FSH levels rise about ten times more, and LH levels about four times more, than those in younger women.[3] This rise is related to an increased pituitary production rate as the metabolic clearance rate of serum FSH and LH are not much different before and after menopause.[4] Episodic secretion continues for both LH and FSH. The pulses of serum FSH are greater in menopausal women than in women during the menstrual cycle. The frequency of the pulses is the same as previously, at 60- to 90-minute intervals. It is the variation in the magnitude of the pulses that accounts for the elevation of basal levels in menopause.[5]

Factors responsible for the selective rise of serum FSH prior to menopause are not really known. The presence of increased serum FSH and normal LH may indicate that a differential regulation exists for gonadotropin secretion; it may be that the ovarian hormone inhibin (which inhibits serum FSH), produced by the granulosa cells, is secreted in lesser amounts with advancing age.[1] The role of follicular function in regulating FSH secretion is evidenced by the observation that plasma FSH is elevated whenever ovarian follicles are absent (e.g., in Turner's syndrome). This selective rise in serum FSH is so characteristic that this hormone has been chosen as the marker of menopause. The upper normal limit has been set at 40 IU/L[6] and any value over that is diagnostic of ovarian failure.

The rise of serum FSH and LH is also related to the increased output of gonadotropin releasing hormone (GnRH) by the hypothalamus, which is similarly deprived of the negative feedback of estrogens. The secretory activity of GnRH neurons is pulsatile. Catecholamines and neuropeptides appear to play a role in regulation of the amplitude and frequency of the pulses; however, these are also under the influence of the ovarian steroids estradiol and progesterone.[7] There is some debate as to whether in menopause there is a change in sensitivity of the hypothalamus and pituitary to estrogen negative and positive feedback. Whether the estrogen-binding capacity of the brain and pituitary is altered with increasing age remains unanswered.

The opioid peptides are preponderant in the control of the hypothalamic-pituitary function. During reproductive years, opioids like β–endorphins exert a tonic inhibition on GnRH release, which is manifested by a suppressive effect in LH secretion.[8] However the suppressive effect, along with the antagonistic effect of naloxone, is manifested only in a high estrogen and progesterone milieu. As this inhibitory influence is ovarian steroid dependent, the administration during menopause of β-endorphin or naloxone has no effect on LH levels.[9] It is then postulated that the high levels of gonadotrophin, in the absence of gonadal steroid feedback, may be related to a diminished opioid inhibition of GnRH release.

GnRH exerts its action by binding to specific receptors in hypophyseal gonadotropes, which stimulates the synthesis and secretion of FSH and LH. Contrary to the unresponsiveness of the postmenopausal ovary to gonadotropins, the hypothalamic-pituitary axis is intact in menopausal women.[10]

Catecholamines also play a significant role in the control of GnRH secretion. The hypothalamus is richly innervated by catecholaminergic fibres. Among the many neurotransmitters identified in the brain, the best known are norepinephrine and dopamine (catecholamines), and serotonin (indolamine). They are believed to be those with the greatest influence on the hypothalamic-pituitary function. Their release and their action are controlled by various mechanisms, such as the degree of re-uptake by the presynaptic terminals, the inhibition by monoamine oxydase (MAO) and catechol-o-methyl-transferase (COMT), and the availability of receptors at the pre- and postsynaptic sites.[11] This regulatory system appears to be modified by various hormones, among which are estrogen and progesterone. Depending on the modification, there will be an increase or a decrease of GnRH secretion by the hypothalamus.

Catechol estrogens are formed by alterations of the A ring of the steroid nucleus, with hydroxylation at the 2 or 4 position. The major metabolite is 2-hydroxy-estrone, and is considered to be the most abundant catechol estrogen in humans. Catechol estrogens are weakly estrogenic, and have a very short half-life. Because of their extraordinarily rapid rate of clearance, it is unlikely that they produce any physiological effect on estrogen receptors or catecholamines, and their importance as circulating estrogens is limited.[12] However, they may have a very important local effect where they are produced, in the hypothalamus, through competitive inhibition of the enzymes tyrosine hydroxylase and COMT. They modulate synthesis and degradation of catecholamines, thereby influencing the production rate of GnRH.[13]

The mechanism responsible for the initiation of the climacteric symptoms such as hot flushes and sleep disturbances is not known. However, it has been proposed that neuroendocrinologic factors, such as changes in catecholamines (perhaps from decreased estrogens), or decline in neurotransmitter activity, may be involved.[14] Catecholamines are thought to play an important role in modulating hypothalamic-pituitary function. Whether aging is associated with an alteration or a deficiency in catecholamine metabolism remains uncertain. Furthermore, ovarian hormones may influence catecholamines in the central nervous system. It has been shown that, in the hypothalamus, castration brings an increase in the concentration of norepinephrine, and a decrease in that of dopamine, along with an increase in the activity of tyrosine hydroxylase (the rate-limiting enzyme in catecholamine synthesis) and in the turnover rate of norepinephrine.[15,16] In summary, the changes observed in the hypothalamus related to estrogen withdrawal point to an increase of the norepinephrine to dopamine ratio that is independent of the aging process.[3]

References

1. Sherman B.M., J.H. West, S.G. Korenman, "The menopausal transition: analysis of LH, FSH, estradiol, and progesterone concentrations during menstrual cycles of older women," *J. Clin. Endocrinol. Metab.* 1976, 42: 629-636.

2. Sherman B.M., S.G. Korenman, "Hormonal characteristics of the human menstrual cycle throughout reproductive life," *J. Clin. Invest.* 1975, 55: 699-706.

3. Yen S.S.C.,"The biology of menopause," *J. Reprod. Med.* 1977, 18: 287-296.

4. Scaglia H, M. Medina, A.L. Pinto-Ferreira *et al.*, "Pituitary LH and FSH secretion and responsiveness in women of old age," *Acta Endocrinol.* 1976, 81: 673-679.

5. Yen S.S.C., C.C. Tsai, F. Naftolin *et al.*, "Pulsatile patterns of gonadotropin release in subjects with and without ovarian function," *J. Clin. Endocrinol.* 1972, 34: 671.

6. Goldenberg R.L., J.M. Grodin, D. Radbard *et al.*, "Gonadotropins in women with amenorrhea," *Am. J. Obstet. Gynecol.* 1973, 116: 1003-1012.

7. Yen S.S.C, "Neuroendocrine regulation of gonadotropin and prolactin secretion in women: disorders in reproduction," Vaitukaitis J.L. (ed): *Clinical Reproductive Neuroendocrinology*, Elsevier Biomedical Press, New York, 1982: 137-175.

8. Ropert J.F., M.E. Quigley, S.S.C. Yen, "Endogenous opiates modulate pulsatile luteinizing hormone release in humans," *J. Clin. Endocrinol. Metab.* 1981; 52: 583-585.

9. Reid R.L., M.E. Quigley, S.S.C Yen, "The disappearance of opiodergic regulation of gonadotropin secretion in postmenopausal women," *J. Clin. Endocrinol. Metab.* 1983, 57: 1107-1110.

10. Wentz A.C., G.S. Jones, L. Rocco, "Gonadotropin responses following luteinizing hormone releasing hormone administration in normal subjects," *Obstet. Gynecol.* 1975, 45: 239-246.

11. Yen S.S.C., "Neuroendocrine control of hypophyseal function," S.S.C. Yen and R.B Jaffe (eds), *Reproductive Endocrinology, Physiology, Pathophysiology, and Clinical Management*, 2nd, Saunders, Philadelphia, 1986: 33-74.

12. Merriam G.R., D.D. Brandon, S. Kone *et al.*, "Rapid metabolic clearance of the catechol estrogen 2-hydroxyestrone," *J. Clin. Endocrinol. Metab.* 1980, 51: 1211-1213.

13. Fishman J., B. Norton, "Brain catecholestrogens: formation and possible function," *Adv. Biosci.* 1975, 15: 123-131.

14. Finch C.E., "Neuroendocrine mechanisms and aging," *Fed. Proc.* 1973, 38: 178-183.

15. Donoso A.O., F.J.E. Stefano, A.M. Biscardi *et al.*, "Effects of castration on hypothalamic catecholamines," *Am. J. Physiol.* 1967, 212: 737-739.

16. Anton-Tay F, R.J. Wurtman, "Norepinephrine turnover in the rat brain after gonadectomy," *Science* 1968, 159: 1245

3. The Postmenopausal Ovary and Steroid Metabolism

Human ovaries have two functions that are closely related during reproductive life:
- cyclic release of oocytes
- production of steroid hormones

During this period, cyclic and repetitive changes in estrogen and progesterone secretion are integrated with follicle maturation, ovulation, and corpus luteum formation and regression.

During the climacteric and menopause, gradual morphologic changes occur within the ovary. These changes produce a gradual decline in gametogenic and steroidogenic functions.

Ovarian Morphology

During adult life, the ovary consists of a predominant outer layer or cortex covered by surface epithelium (mesothelium) and containing connective tissue, follicular tissue, stromal cells, large blood vessels, lymphatics, and nerves.

During the climacteric period, anovulation and atretic follicles will predominate the ovarian morphology which becomes mainly corticomedullary stroma. The ovary in the postmenopausal period loses half its weight to 5 g or less due to volumetric decrease, involutional vascular changes, deposition of pigment, cortical fibrosis, and declining steroidogenesis.[1,2] However, the ovaries remain active during the postmenopausal years even if they are depleted of their follicular reserve. Atretic follicles, cystic follicles, and luteinized follicular cysts may remain even 10 years after menopause.[3] Fibrous corpora albicantia with a well-preserved microvascular blood supply may persist into the eighth and ninth decades of life.[4]

After menopause, there is an increase in the incidence of cortical granulomata and surface epithelium cysts, and a predominance of hilar cells in 83% of ovaries, especially in women more than 70 years old. Stromal luteinization and proliferation is associated with clinical signs of androgen hypersecretion[5] and appears to be a function of parity, suggesting a pathogenic role for gonadotropins.

Correlation Between Structure and Function of the Ovaries

Signals from the brain and pituitary to the ovaries stimulate the production of estrogens. Estrogens have an essential action on tissues of the female reproductive tract and influence metabolism in the liver, fat, bone, and vascular system. Substances such as progesterone, protein binding globulins, glucocorticoids, and androgens help to regulate estrogen actions.

Postmenopausal Estrogen Production

During the years of reproduction, there are two sources of estrogen production: the major source is the secretion of 17β-estradiol by granulosa cells of the ovarian follicles, and the other source involves extraglandular aromatization of plasma androstenedione. During menopause, with the loss of responsiveness and the decrease in the number of granulosa cells, the cyclical secretion of estradiol and progesterone ceases. However, a small amount of testosterone and androstenedione are still produced by the ovaries after menopause. These androgens, in the presence of declining estrogens, may lead to hirsutism. With advancing age, the adrenal secretion of androstenedione does not decline. Androstenedione is converted to estrone in peripheral and stromal tissues such as bone, fat, muscle, brain, and skin. This conversion accounts for most, if not all, the estrogens produced during menopause.[6] Although a reduction in the production of androstenedione from 3 mg/day to 1.5 mg/day is observed in menopause, this decline is related almost exclusively to a decreased secretion of androstenedione by menopausal ovaries.

Estrone is a weak estrogen which is converted to estradiol in many tissues. The usual production of estrone by non-obese postmenopausal women has been estimated to be 40 µg/day. The conversion rate is about 2.8% and accounts for almost all the estradiol produced in menopausal women.[6,7] Estrone does not bind to sex hormone binding globulin (SHBG) and binds only loosely to albumin.[8,9] Consequently, it has a more rapid clearance rate than estradiol. When the daily production rate of estrone exceeds 75 µg because of multiple factors such as age, obesity, liver disease, hyperthyroidism, compensated congestive heart failure, starvation, non-endocrine tumours, and endocrine tumours of the ovaries, uterine bleeding may occur.[10]

The amount of estrogens produced by postmenopausal women correlates with increasing body weight. Many studies have demonstrated that adipose tissue and adipocytes contain the enzyme aromatase which is responsible for the conversion of androstenedione to estrogens, but conversion is also related to dietary, metabolic, and genetic factors. Endometrial hyperplasia and carcinoma of the endometrium have been long associated with high estrogen levels and excessive body weight.[11] Severe osteoporosis is often seen in thin women with lower estrogen production. Androgen and estrogen levels have been compared in postmenopausal women with endometrial cancer (obese) and those with osteoporosis (thin). No differences in androstenedione and testosterone levels were noted, but total estrone and estradiol levels in obese women were significantly higher than in thin women; the amount of free estradiol was 2.5- to 3-fold higher in obese women.[11]

Bioavailability: Hormone Binding and Transport

During menopause, the main circulating estrogen is estrone, an estrogen with weaker affinity for estrogen receptors than estradiol. Serum levels average 20 to 60 pg/mL (70-200 pmol/L). However, estradiol is still present in the blood at a concentration of 15 to 25 pg/mL (50 to 90 pmol/L) or less. Progesterone is measured at 0.5 ng/mL (1.5 nmol/L) or less and comes entirely from the adrenals (Table 1).

Only the free fraction of steroid in plasma is thought to be able to enter target cells and exert biological effects. 17β-estradiol is converted from estrone in the tissues but only 5% will eventually enter the blood stream. One of the major means of regulating the free concentration of estrogens is the concentration of sex hormone binding globulin (SHBG) and albumin.

Table 1:
Plasma sex hormone concentrations in pre- and postmenopausal women*

Hormone Concentration	Premenopausal		Postmenopausal
	Minimum	Maximum	
Estradiol (pg/mL)	50-60	300-500	5-25
Estrone (pg/mL)	30-40	150-300	20-60
Progesterone (ng/mL)	0.5-1.0	10-20	0.5
Androstenedione (ng/mL)		1.0-2.0	0.3-1.0
Testosterone (ng/mL)		0.3-0.8	0.1-0.5

* D.R. Mishell, Jr. (ed). *Menopause: Physiology and Pharmacology*, Year Book Medical Publishers Inc., Chicago, 1987: 48.

Sex Hormone Binding Globulin

Estradiol, testosterone, and 5α-dihydrotestosterone bind SHBG competitively with affinities in ratios of approximately 0.4:1:3.[12,13] Androstenedione, dihydroepiandrosterone, estrone, estrone sulphate, and estriol are poorly bound by SHBG. Albumin has higher affinities for estrone, estrone sulphate, and estriol.[14,15] Approximately 38% of estradiol is bound to SHBG, 60% to albumin, and 2 to 3% is free in the circulation.[16] SHBG, therefore, influences hormone availability, metabolism, and exposure to end organ receptors. The concentration of SHBG may be severely depressed in obese postmenopausal women.[17] Consequently, increases in the percentage of free estradiol[17-19] and in the availability of plasma estrogens to target tissues are observed.

Estrone Sulphate Pool

Estrone sulphate is formed by conjugation within the liver. In the blood, estrone sulphate is loosely bound to albumin and serves as an inactive reservoir of precursor for the formation of estradiol and estrone. Estrone sulphate may be hydrolyzed to estrone at a rate of 21% and be converted to estradiol at a rate of 1.4%.

Receptor Binding or Cellular Mechanisms in Postmenopausal Women

Steroids diffuse into target cells and interact with specific gene regulatory sites on DNA in the nucleus to modulate messenger RNA synthesis.

There is no special mechanism of intracellular binding to receptors in post-menopausal women. However, the positive cooperativity in estradiol binding could explain why very low-doses of various estrogen medications may elicit biological effects out of proportion in some postmenopausal women. Measurement of total plasma estradiol alone cannot accurately reflect the impact on target tissues since only small increases in intracellular estradiol levels sometimes activate estrogen receptors.

References

1. Nicosia, S.V., "Morphological changes of the human ovary throughout life," G.B. Serra (ed), *The Ovary*, Raven Press, New York, 1983: 57-82.

2. Lang W.R., G.E. Aponte, "Gross and microscopic anatomy of the aged female reproductive organs," *Clin. Obstet. Gynecol.* 1967, 10: 454-465.

3. Boss J.H., R.E. Scully, K.H. Wegner *et al.*, "Structural Variations in the Adult Ovary – Clinical Significance," *Obstet. Gynecol.* 1965, 25: 747-764.

4. Thung P.J., "Aging changes in the ovary," G.H. Bourne (ed), *Structural Aspects of Aging*, Hafner, New York, 1961: 109-142.

5. Laffargue P., L. Benkoël, F. Laffargue *et al.*, "Ultrastructural and enzyme histochemical study of ovarian hilar cells in women and their relationships with sympathetic nerves," *Hum. Pathol.* 1978, 9: 649-659.

6. Grodin J.M., P.K. Siiteri, P.C. MacDonald, "Source of estrogen production in postmenopausal women," *J. Clin. Endocrinol. Metab.* 1973, 36: 207-214.

7. Vermeulen A., "The hormonal activity of postmenopausal ovary," *J. Clin. Endocrinol. Metab.* 1976, 42: 247-253.

8. Longcope C., "Metabolic clearance and blood production rates of estrogens in postmenopausal women," *Am. J. Obstet. Gynecol.* 1971, 111: 778-781.

9. Longcope C., J.F. Tait, "Validity of metabolic clearance and interconversion rates of estrone and 17β- estradiol in normal adults," *J. Clin. Endocrinol. Metab.* 1971; 32: 481-490.

10. MacDonald P.C., J.M. Grodin, P.K. Siiteri, "The utilization of plasma androstenedione for estrone production in women," C. Gual and F.J.G. Ebling (eds), *Progress in Endocrinology: Proceedings of the Third International Congress of Endocrinology*, Excerpta Medica Foundation, Amsterdam, 1969: 770-776.

11. Laufer L.R., B.J. Davidson, R.K. Ross *et al*, "Physical characteristics and sex hormone levels in patients with osteoporotic hip fractures or endometrial cancer," *Am. J. Obstet. Gynecol.* 1983, 145: 585-590.

12. Anderson D.C., "The role of sex hormone binding globulin in health and disease," V.H.T. James, M. Serio and G. Giusti (eds), *The Endocrine Function of the Human Ovary*, Academic Press, London, 1976: 141-158.

13. Moll, G.W., R.L. Rosenfield and J.H. Helke, "Estradiol-testosterone binding interactions and free plasma estradiol under physiological condition," *J. Clin. Endocrinol. Metab.* 1981, 52: 868-874.

14. Rosenthal H.E., E. Pietrzak, W.R. Slaunwhite *et al.*, "Binding of estrone sulfate in human plasma," *J. Clin. Endocrinol. Metab.* 1972, 34: 805-813.

15. Murphy B.P., "Protein binding and radioassays of estrogens and progestins," R.O. Greep, E.B. Astwood (eds): *Handbook of Physiology*, Section 7: Endocrinology, Vol. 2, Female reproductive system, part 1, American Physiological Society, Washington, DC, 1973: 631-642.

16. Wu C.-H., T. Motohashi, H.A. Abdel-Rahman *et al.*, "Free and protein-bound plasma estradiol-17β during the menstrual cycle," *J. Clin. Endocrinol. Metab.* 1976, 43: 436-445.

17. Nisker J.A., G.L. Hammond, B.J. Davidson *et al.*, "Serum sex hormone-binding globulin capacity and the percentage of free estradiol in postmenopausal women with and without endometrial carcinoma. A new biochemical basis for the association between obesity and endometrial carcinoma," *Am. J. Obstet. Gynecol.* 1980, 138: 637-642.

18. Siiteri P.K., "Review of studies on estrogen biosynthesis in the human," *Cancer Res.* 1982, 42(suppl): 3269s-3273s.

19. Siiteri P.K., J.T. Murai, G.L. Hammond *et al.*, "The serum transfer of steroid hormones," *Recent Prog. Horm. Res.* 1982, 38: 457-510.

4. Physiologic Changes of Menopause

Hot Flushes

Hot flushes are considered to be one of the signs of menopause, although they may be observed during the perimenopausal years. They are experienced by up to 80% of women undergoing natural or surgical menopause. The majority of women with hot flushes will present with them for more than a year, and almost half of women for up to five or ten years after cessation of menstruation.[1]

Excellent description of the hot flush has been provided.[2] The first indication of its imminence is described as a sensation of pressure in the head, comparable to a headache. This feeling is progressive in intensity and culminates in the actual hot flush which starts in the head and neck areas and passes like a wave over the entire body. It is described as a hot or burning sensation, and is usually followed by sweating in various degrees, more intense in the head, the neck and the upper chest, and less pronounced on the cheeks and legs. The entire episode is transient, lasting 2 to 5 minutes, and may be followed by a chill and shivering.

The physiology of the hot flush has been investigated mainly in the last 15 years. Molnar first described temperature changes on skin surfaces and internal orifices.[3,4] Other studies documented the characteristic changes in finger and central temperature, and skin resistance.[5-7] Skin temperature was recorded over the dorsum of the proximal phalanx of the non-dominant hand, and showed an average increase of 2.7°C (1.4 to 4.9), with a mean duration of 8.3 minutes for the increase phase and of 23 minutes for the decrease phase, for a total duration of 31 minutes. The subjective flushing had a mean duration of 2.3 minutes (with a range of 35 seconds to 5 minutes), and that of perspiration was 2.1 minutes. In two thirds of the subjects, the objective flushing was noticed before the onset of the temperature elevation.[5]

A decrease in core temperature has been observed following the hot flush as measured by a probe placed in the external auditory canal, and is in the range of 0.2°C.[6] The beginning of this decline has been observed 3.1 minutes after the start of the rise in finger temperature.[13] Skin resistance was assessed by passing a current between two electrodes placed 4 cm apart on the sternum, and showed a decrease during the flush. This measurement is believed to be the most sensitive indicator of the hot flush as it has been associated with it in almost all the episodes;[7] it is always the first one registered, and is followed by a rise in finger temperature and then a decrease in central temperature. Pulse rate is increased by 9 to 20 beats per minute; no change in blood pressure is observed.[8] There is a rapid rise in blood flow to the hands, which may be observed even before the perception of the flush.[9] Actually, the flush is perceived only while the skin temperature is increasing, and is out of proportion to the rise in temperature, which is minimal. The heightened perception may be related to the rate of temperature change as well as to the increase itself.[8]

As the typical hot flush also occurs at night, it has been observed that women awake before any characteristic changes associated with the flush occur.[10] There is a decrease in REM sleep and in sleep latency in untreated menopausal women compared to those taking estrogen.[11] It appears obvious why menopausal women afflicted with frequent hot flushes are subjected to sleep deprivation, and complain of nervousness, irritability, lack of concentration, and generally speaking diminished quality of life.

The relationship between hot flushes and hormonal changes has been examined in several studies using a multiple sampling technique.[12-15] Hot flushes are always associated with a pulsatile release of luteinizing hormone (LH), whereas thyroid stimulating hormone (TSH) and prolactin (PRL) remain unchanged. There appears to be no correlation with follicle stimulating hormone (FSH).[16] The release of LH pulses occurs simultaneously with the flush, and does not precede it; the minimal level of serum LH is measured shortly after the peak of finger temperature. The LH pulse cannot be the cause of the flush, since flushes occur in women following hypophysectomy; they also occur in women where the pituitary has been desensitized by a potent gonadotropin releasing hormone (GnRH) analog: the LH pulses are abolished, but the flushes are still present.[17]

A significantly lower level of estradiol along with a lower mean body weight has been found in women complaining of severe hot flushes as compared to women who are asymptomatic.[19] The lack of symptoms in the latter group has been related to a greater peripheral aromatization of androgen precursors. However, during the flush no significant change in peripheral estrogens has been documented.[15]

Growth hormone was found significantly increased at 20 minutes after the rise in finger temperature, and adrenocorticotropic hormone (ACTH) at 5 minutes.[15] Maximal increase in cortisol was noted at 15 minutes, along with a rise of dehydroepiandrosterone (DHEA), androstenedione, compound F, and progesterone, which is believed to be derived from increased adrenal activity following the hot flush[18]. The release of ACTH from the pituitary is thought to be associated with actual cooling of the hypothalamus, as the phenomenon has been described in the goat.[20] Indeed, a loss of peripheral heat during the hot flush brings a drop in core temperature beginning 3.1 minutes after the onset of temperature elevation.[6]

Although the etiology of the hot flush is not known with certainty, it appears that it is related to a sudden change in central thermoregulation. It has been proposed that the flush is initiated by a sudden downward setting of the central thermostat, and this event would coincide with the aura preceding the flush by about 45 seconds.[6] In response, a series of physiological changes is initiated promoting heat loss and aiming to bring the body temperature back to the new set point. The hot flush is observed, and accompanied by a significant increase of growth hormone and LH. The release of both hormones is thought to be mediated in the hypothalamus by a neurotransmitter, mainly norepinephrine.[21,22] It has been suggested that, in the estrogen-deprived hypothalamus, an increase in norepinephrine activity would stimulate the release of both growth hormone and LH, and at the same time activate thermo-regulatory centres situated nearby.[14] These two events would be explained by a common underlying hypothalamic endocrine disorder.

The role of the opioid peptides also has been considered in the etiology of the hot flush. In the normal premenopausal woman, a naloxone infusion results in increased LH pulsatile release and LH levels.[23] This finding suggests that endogenous opiates are inhibitors of gonadotropin release. However, during menopause a naloxone infusion fails to augment gonadotropin release, and has no effect whatsoever on the number of hot flushes, the level of LH or FSH, and the variation of the gonadotropin pulses.[24,25] It appears that the hypothalamic secretion of β-endorphins is estrogen-dependent, and that the level of these peptides may be so low in an estrogen- and progesterone-deprived environment that they have no role in controlling gonadotropin secretion.

In conclusion, the hot flush appears to originate in the estrogen-deprived hypothalamus, where some neuroendocrine imbalance triggers the thermo-regulatory centre; this event may be mediated by a neurotransmitter, possibly norepinephrine, but more data need to be gathered to support this speculation.

References

1. Anderson E., S. Hamburger, J.H. Liu *et al.*, "Characteristics of menopausal women seeking assistance," *Am. J. Obstet. Gynecol.* 1987, 156: 428-433.

2. Judd H.L., "Menopause and postmenopause," R.C. Benson (ed): *Current Obstetric and Gynecologic Diagnosis and Treatment*, Lange Medical Publications, Los Altos, California, 1984: 570-589.

3. Molnar G.W., "Body temperatures during menopausal hot flashes," *J. Appl. Physiol.* 1975, 38: 499-503.

4. Idem: "Investigation of hot flashes by ambulatory monitoring," *Am. J. Physiol.* 1979, 237: R306-R310.

5. Meldrum D.R., I.M. Shamonki, A.M. Frumar *et al.*, "Elevations in skin temperature of the finger as an objective index of postmenopausal hot flashes: standardization of the technique," *Am. J. Obstet. Gynecol.* 1979, 135: 713-717.

6. Tataryn I.V., P. Lomax, J.G. Bajorek *et al.*, "Postmenopausal hot flushes: a disorder of thermoregulation," *Maturitas* 1980, 2: 101-107.

7. Tataryn I.V., P. Lomax, D.R. Meldrum *et al.*, "Objective techniques for the assessment of postmenopausal hot flashes," *Obstet. Gynecol.* 1981, 57: 340-344.

8. Sturdee D.W., K.A. Wilson, E. Pipili *et al.*, "Physiological aspects of menopausal hot flush. *Br. Med. J.* 1978, 2: 79-80.

9. Ginsburg J, J. Swinhoe, B. O'Reilly, "Cardiovascular responses during the menopausal hot flush," *Br. J. Obstet. Gynaecol.* 1981, 88: 925-930.

10. Erlik Y., I.V. Tataryn, D.R. Meldrum *et al.*, "Association of waking episodes with menopausal hot flushes," *JAMA* 1981, 245: 1741-1744.

11. Schiff I, Q. Regestein, D. Tulchinsky *et al.*, "Effects of estrogens on sleep and psychological state of hypogonadal women," *JAMA* 1979, 242: 2405-2407.

12. Casper R.F., S.S.C. Yen, M.M. Wilkes, "Menopausal flushes: a neuroendocrine link with pulsatile luteinizing hormone secretion," *Science* 1979, 205: 823-825.

13. Tataryn I.V., D.R. Meldrum, K.H. Lu *et al.*, "LH, FSH and skin temperature during the menopausal hot flash," *J. Clin. Endocrinol. Metab.* 1979, 49: 152-154.

14. Meldrum D.R., J.D. Defazio, Y. Erlik *et al.*, "Pituitary hormones during the menopausal hot flash," *Obstet. Gynecol.* 1984, 64: 752-756.

15. Meldrum D.R., I.V. Tataryn, A.M. Frumar *et al.*, "Gonadotropins, estrogens, and adrenal steroids during the menopausal hot flash," *J. Clin. Endocrinol. Metab.* 1980, 50: 685-689.

16. Mashchak C.A., O.A. Kletzky, R. Artal *et al.*, "The relation of physiological changes to subjective symptoms in postmenopausal women with and without hot flushes," *Maturitas* 1984, 6: 301-308.

17. Casper R.F., S.S.C. Yen, "Menopausal flushes: effect of pituitary gonadotropin desensitization by a potent luteinizing hormone-releasing factor agonist," *J. Clin. Endocrinol. Metab.* 1981, 53: 1056-1058.

18. Kronenberg F., L.J. Cote, D.M. Linkie *et al.*, "Menopausal hot flashes: thermoregulatory, cardiovascular, and circulating catecholamine and LH changes," *Maturitas* 1984, 6: 31-43.

19. Erlik Y., D.R. Meldrum, H.L. Judd, "Estrogen levels in postmenopausal women with hot flashes," *Obstet. Gynecol.* 1982, 59: 403-407.

20. Williams D.D., P. Marques, P. Illner *et al.*, "Endocrine responses to cooling of the hypothalamus in goats. Drugs, biogenic amines and body temperature," K.E. Cooper, P. Lomax, E. Schönbaum (eds), *Proceedings of the Third Symposium on the Pharmacology of Thermoregulation*, Karger, Basel, 1977: 62-65.

21. Weiner R.F., W.F. Ganong, "Role of brain monoamines and histamine in regulation of anterior pituitary secretion," *Physiol. Rev.* 1978, 58: 905-976.

22. Bhattacharya A.N., D.J. Dierschke, T. Yamaji *et al.*, "The pharmacologic blockade of the circhoral mode of LH secretion in the ovariectomized rhesus monkey," *Endocrinol.* 1972, 90: 778-786.

23. Quigley M.E., S.S.C. Yen, "The role of endogenous opiates on LH secretion during the menstrual cycle," *J. Clin. Endocrinol. Metab.* 1980, 51: 179-181

24. DeFazio J., C. Verheugen, R. Chetkowski *et al.*, "The effects of naloxone on hot flashes and gonadotropin secretion in postmenopausal women," *J. Clin. Endocrinol. Metab.* 1984, 58: 578-581.

25. Tulandi T., R.A. Kinch, H. Guyda *et al.*, "Effect of naloxone on menopausal flushes, skin temperature, and luteinizing hormone secretion," *Am. J. Obstet. Gynecol.* 1985, 151: 277-280.

Genitourinary System Changes

The lower one third of the vagina, the vulva, urethra, and trigone of the bladder have a common embryological origin. They are all rich in estrogen receptors, as is the vasculature of these areas. In the presence of estrogen deficiency, blood flow to the vulva and vagina decreases by approximately 60%. Changes in the lower genitourinary tract as a result of estrogen deprivation consist of thinning and atrophy of the sub-dermal layers of the vulva and loss of vaginal rugae. There is decreased vaginal lubrication during intercourse as a result of the reduced blood supply to the vaginal barrel. In addition, there is loss of elasticity, shortening, and narrowing of the vagina which may result in dyspareunia. The vagina is easily traumatized and bleeding after intercourse is common. Thinning and flattening of the vaginal epithelium, with resultant reduction in the production of lactic acid, leads to increased alkalinity of the vaginal secretions, irritation, and infection.

Similar atrophic changes in the lower urinary tract may result in the "urethral syndrome," which consists of recurrent abacterial urethritis. The most common symptom of this syndrome is nocturia. Narrowing of the distal segment of the urethra may lead to outflow obstruction. Other symptoms include post-voidal dribbling and stress incontinence.

Dermatological Changes

Changes occur in the skin and connective tissue as a result of estrogen deprivation. There is a decrease in intercellular fluid content[1] which results in thinning and atrophy of the sub-dermal layers as well as a decrease in sebaceous and sweat gland activity. This increases the sensitivity of the skin to temperature and humidity. There is a loss of pubic, axillary, and scalp hair.

There are also changes in collagen content of connective tissue as a result of aging. Type 1 collagen accounts for 90% of body collagen and is the major connective tissue protein, found in skin, bone, and other tissues. Serious attention has been given to the possibility that measurement of collagen content of the skin may help to identify the patient at risk for early progressive osteoporosis.[2] In a prospective study of postmenopausal women, it has been shown that skin collagen declines irrespective of the age of the woman in the postmenopausal years.[3] This decline can be arrested by hormone replacement therapy. However, in a more recent study, it was shown that women with low skin collagen levels respond to estrogen with a greater increase than do women with higher skin collagen levels and who in addition are closer to menopause. There is, moreover, an optimum level beyond which very little improvement occurs.[2]

It has been shown that skin exposed regularly to ultraviolet light will lose water and elasticity, changes which are not necessarily reversed by hormonal therapy.[4]

The presence of subcutaneous fat has certain benefits in the menopausal woman. Androstenedione is metabolized in fat to estrone which may promote a longer interval before complete estrogen deprivation is apparent. Also, the risk of osteoporotic fractures is not only reduced but relegated to a more advanced age.

Voice changes have been associated with the postmenopausal period.[5] A reduction in the upper register and a loss of timbre was found – not serious except to someone who is a singer. Further information was provided by a study carried out at Marquette University, Milwaukee.[6] During middle age (45 to 55 years), women produce a significantly lower low frequency pitch than do young (25 to 35) or old (70 to 80 women). This enhanced low frequency capability of middle age is not carried into old age. In old age, there is also a loss of ability to produce high frequencies and therefore there is a reduction in range of pitch. This phenomenon occurs later in life and not as an immediate consequence of menopause. These changes may be the result of the passage of time, wear and tear factors, and changing levels of hormones.[6] They are examples of the many changes associated with aging and estrogen withdrawal which, while not a serious health hazard, mark the passage of time.

References

1.   Branwood A.W., "The fibroblast," *Int. Rev. Connect. Tiss. Res.* 1963, 1: 1-28.

2.   Brincat M., T.W. Yeun, J.W.W. Studd *et al.*, "Response of skin thickness and metacarpal index to estradiol therapy in postmenopausal women," *Obstet. Gynecol.* 1987, 70: 538-541.

3.   Brincat M, C.F. Moniz, J.W.W. Studd *et al.*, "Sex hormones and skin collagen content in postmenopausal women," *Br. Med. J.* 1983, 287: 1337-1338.

4.   Barbo D.M., "The postmenopausal woman," *Med. Clin. N. Am.* 1987, 71(1): 1-152

5.   Van Keep P.A., A.A. Haspel, "*Estrogen Therapy During the Climacteric and Afterwards,*" Excerpta Medica, Amsterdam, 1977.

6.   Linville S.E., "Maximum phonational frequency range capabilities of women's voices with advancing age," *Folia Phoniatr.*, 1987, 39: 297-301.

Changes in Lipid Metabolism

It is important to note that serum cholesterol fractions vary with age and are different between men and women.[1] In young women, plasma low density lipoprotein-cholesterol (LDL-C) concentrations and total cholesterol levels are lower than in men of similar age. In men, there is a steady increase in LDL-C until age 40 and a tendency to plateau thereafter. In women, this fraction slowly increases until age 45 but markedly increases between 45 and 55 years of age corresponding to the period of menopause. Over the age of 50, mean low density lipoprotein (LDL) concentrations in women exceed those of men. High density lipoprotein-cholesterol (HDL-C) is always higher in women than in men at any age. However, there is a slow decrease in HDL-C after age 50 in women. The ratio of LDL-C/HDL-C (atherogenic index) is thus rapidly increasing at the time of menopause.

Menopause, whether surgically induced at an early age or biologically achieved during the middle years, is also associated with a change in the lipoprotein moieties and cholesterol transfer mechanisms.[2] The levels of other lipoprotein lipids also increase, including very low density lipoproteins (VLDL) and intermediate density lipoproteins (IDL), further contributing to athero-genesis.[3] This redistribution of cholesterol into the LDL fraction appears to result from the gradual fall in circulating levels of estrogen. Several, but not all, authors have also found a significant increase in triglyceride concentration in the postmenopause[4-8] and some have related it to age rather than ovarian failure.

There is no consensus on the effects of ovarian failure on individual lipoproteins. Two studies[9,10] reported no change in high density lipoproteins but a rise in low density lipoproteins after menopause; another study[6] found lower high density lipoprotein levels. Finally, it has been observed that serum cholesterol and triglycerides are significantly higher in postmenopausal groups and also increase with advancing postmenopausal age,[11] HDL-C levels may be increased and LDL-C may be decreased in menopause by estrogens.[12,13] High density lipoprotein (HDL) serves to accelerate lecithin/cholesterol acyl transferase activity, promoting the transfer of cholesterol from tissue to plasma and facilitating its subsequent entrance to the liver for metabolism and excretion.

References

1. LaRosa J.C., "Women, lipoproteins and cardiovascular disease risk," *Can. J. Cardiol.* 1990, 6(suppl B): 23B-29B.

2. Hjortland M.C., P.M. McNamara, W.B. Kannel, "Some atherogenic concomitants of menopause: the Framingham Study," *Am. J. Epidemiol.* 1976, 103: 304-311.

3. Canadian Lipoprotein Conference Ad Hoc Committee on Guidelines for Dyslipoproteinemias, "Guidelines for the detection of high-risk lipoprotein profiles and the treatment of dyslipoproteinemias," *Can. Med. Assoc. J.* 1990, 142: 1371-1382.

4. Lindquist O., "Influence of menopause on ischaemic heart disease and its risk factors on bone mineral content," *Acta. Obstet. Gynecol. Scand.* 1982, suppl 110: 1-21.

5. Paterson M.E.L., D.W. Sturdee, B. Moore, "The effect of menopausal status and sequential mestranol and norethisterone on serum cholesterol, triglyceride and electrophoretic lipoprotein patterns," *Br. J. Obstet. Gynaecol.* 1979, 86: 810-815.

6. Notelovitz M, J.C. Gudat, M.D. Ware et al., "Lipids and lipoproteins in women after oophorectomy and the response to oestrogen therapy," *Br. J. Obstet. Gynaecol.* 1983, 90: 171-177.

7. Johansson B.W., L. Kaij, S. Kullander *et al.*, "On some late effects of bilateral oophorectomy in the age range 15-30 years," *Acta. Obstet. Gynecol. Scand.* 1975, 54: 449-461.

8. Hallberg L, A. Svanborg, "Cholesterol, phospholipids and triglycerides in plasma in 50 year-old women," *Acta. Med. Scand.* 1967, 181: 185-194.

9. Kannel W.B., M.C. Hjortland, P.M. McNamara *et al.*, "Menopause and risk of cardiovascular disease: the Framingham Study," *Ann. Int. Med.* 1976, 85: 447-452.

10. Robinson R.W., N. Higano, W.D. Cohen, "Increased incidence of coronary heart disease in women castrated prior to menopause," *AMA Arch. Int. Med.* 1959, 104: 908-913.

11. Bengtsson C., O. Lindquist, "Menopausal effects on risk-factors for ischaemic heart-disease," *Maturitas* 1979, 1: 165-170.

12. Wahl P.W., G.R. Warnick, J.J. Albers *et al.*, "Distribution of lipoprotein, triglyceride and lipoprotein cholesterol in an adult population by age, sex, and hormone use," *Atherosclerosis* 1981, 39: 111-124.

13. Krauss R.M., "Regulation of high density lipoprotein levels," *Med. Clin. N. Am.* 1982, 66: 403-430.

Changes in Carbohydrate Metabolism

Glucose tolerance decreases with advancing age. It is not known if this is the result of hormonal changes or an impairment at the cellular and pancreatic levels associated with advancing age. Menopause does not appear to be diabetogenic in the absence of underlying disease. In postmenopausal women, synthetic and natural estrogen therapy may produce mildly abnormal carbohydrate tolerance but rarely is frank diabetes observed.[1,2] It appears that natural estrogens cause fewer disturbances in carbohydrate metabolism and insulin levels than do synthetic estrogens,[3,4] even if the dosage used is in excess of that normally used for treatment of menopausal symptoms.[5] While the glucose tolerance curves reveal significant differences at some points in the curve,[3,4] it is worthwhile to note that most investigators do not report the development of frank, clinically evident diabetes mellitus in patients using estrogen replacement therapy. The combination of estrogen and progestin may have a synergistic effect on glucose intolerance.[6] Estrogens are therefore not contraindicated in diabetic patients, although it would be prudent to monitor glucose levels at regular intervals.

In the menopausal years, the following have been observed:

- Frank diabetes of the adult type is diagnosed more often and presents itself without the classical symptoms of polyuria, polydipsia, and polyphagia.
- Very often, the presenting symptoms are fatigue, lethargy, obesity, or neuropathy.
- The more serious complications of nephropathy, retinopathy, or ketoacidosis are less frequent.
- The onset of hyperosmolar non-ketotic coma is insidious and may result from changes in mental status and dehydration.

References

1. Gow S., I. MacGillivray, "Metabolic, hormonal and vascular changes after synthetic oestrogen therapy in oophorectomized women," *Br. Med. J.* 1971; 2: 73-77.

2. Notelovitz M., "Metabolic effect of conjugated estrogens (USP) on glucose tolerance," *S. Afr. Med. J.* 1974, 48: 2599-2603.

3. Thom M., S. Chakravarti, D.H. Oram *et al.*, "Effect of hormone replacement therapy on glucose tolerance in postmenopausal women," *Br. J. Obstet. Gynaecol.* 1977, 84: 776-783.

4. Larson-Cohn U., L. Wallentin, "Metabolic and hormonal effects of postmenopausal estrogen replacement treatment. I. Glucose insulin, and human growth hormone levels during oral glucose tolerance tests," *Acta. Endocrinol.* 1977, 86: 583-596.

5. Shahmanesh M., C.H. Bolton, R.C. Feneley *et al.*, "Metabolic effects of estrogen treatment in patients with carcinoma of the prostate. A comparison of stilboestrol and conjugated equine estrogens," *Br. Med. J.* 1973, 2: 512-514

6. Spellacy W.H., W.B. Buhi, S.A. Burk, "The effects of estrogens on carbohydrate metabolism: glucose, insulin and growth hormone studies on 171 women ingesting Premarin, mestranol and ethinyl estradiol for 6 months. *Am. J. Obstet. Gynecol.* 1972, 114: 378-392.

Psychological Transitions Associated with Menopause

Menopause has many dimensions. It acts as a marker of aging; it is predicated on alterations of hormonal patterning with physiological consequence, and it is a time of personal re-evaluation of self in relation to family, workplace, life goals, and sexuality. Many of the emotive states and feelings women are experiencing during this period are a function of adjustment to personal life content, while others are more globally based upon social realities for North American women. Impending old age may elicit fears of aloneness (widowhood), loss of income, loss of autonomy, loss of options in the workplace, loss of life goals never realized.[1]

Medical literature has defined menopause attitudinally as a time of deficiency and decline, implying a disease state needing treatment rather than a physiological function of aging. It is also biased by studies on predominantly white, middle-class women.

A Western consumer culture bases worth on youthfulness, appearance, fertility, and conformity. The achievements and contributions of women in the menopausal age group may be devalued or even dismissed within a profession or workplace, particularly if the workplace is the home. In addition, if cultural devaluation coincides with menopause, it is important to determine, in counselling with the woman, her level of satisfaction and fulfilment in all aspects of her life to better understand her psychological response.

Canada now houses a diverse racial and ethnic population with particular coping skills, transitional life cycle customs and philosophical understandings of aging built on tradition and ritual. Women from cultures in which aging increases personal worth, status, and privilege are seen as confidantes, advisors, decision makers, and leaders. Many cultures view midlife as a healthy time of balance as menopause liberates a woman from the fear of pregnancy, nuisance of birth control, and offers her more leisure time and privacy.[2] It is interesting to note that, in countries where postmenopausal women have a special and important status, there are few menopausal complaints.[3]

Psychological symptoms associated with menopause are many and varied. Nervousness, anxiety, irritability, fatigue, headaches, depression, and sleep disturbances are common complaints. How these psychological symptoms are interrelated, and how much they result from estrogen deprivation, environmental stress, and natural aging, is not clear at present. Certainly, hot flushes are associated with sleep disturbances which in turn can lead to fatigue, irritability, and other symptoms of sleep deprivation. In a study carried out at UCLA, it was found that there was a significant relationship between the occurrence of "flushes" and waking episodes.[4] In another study, complaints of sleep disturbances and insomnia rose as estrogen levels fell.[5] Following these observations, a double-blind controlled study looking at administration of exogenous estrogen on sleep found a significant decrease in wakefulness, frequency of nocturnal awakenings, and an increase in total REM sleep.[6] While interruption of sleep due to hot flushes is inevitable, considerable reductions in the number of waking episodes were noted by all women receiving estrogen therapy. It appears that altered sleep patterns in menopause may act as a stressor which may precipitate any form of psychologic disturbance in the predisposed woman.

More affluent women tend to be in better health and receive more adequate health services. Socioeconomic differences affect older women's quality of shelter, nutrition, social participation, household assistance, and medical care. Psychological factors such as social class and being employed are better predictors of both psychological and related somatic symptoms than (hormonal) menopausal status.[7] A child leaving home is not itself necessarily stressful;[8] rather bereavements and losses are more potent predictors of somatic symptoms.[9,10] Widowhood, divorce, and separation may occur in the perimenopausal or postmenopausal years.

It is erroneous to assume that cessation of menstruation and loss of fertility represents a trauma for all women. Studies of women's psychological adaptation to menopause are based upon those who present to the health care system, whereas the majority of women do not present to the medical community unless they have a problematic symptom complex.

The cessation of menstruation fosters a realization of the aging process. This requires an adjustment in self-definition. The ability to adapt depends upon many factors, including employment history, cultural background, children, socio-economic environment, and education. Women react to menopause in accordance with symptoms experienced, and access and availability of support systems and information which often tend to reflect social and economic status.[11] Medical attitudes which view women as resources in decision making about their personal health care increase self-esteem and empower women. The support provided by her sexual partner, family, and community may be of considerable benefit.

Patterns of anxiety and depressive states have been identified in the self-help movement through women's reporting on the menopausal transition.[12] Five patterns emerge:

- There is a daily episodic "blues" where the person experiences low spirits, reduced drive, and feelings of pessimism. Acknowledgement of these feeling states is helpful. Pharmacotherapy is not warranted.
- Grief (mourning) – often associated with perceived loss (status, employment, life goals) or personal loss (parents, relatives, friends), associated with feelings of guilt, sleep disturbance, and tearfulness. Counselling is beneficial. Pharmacotherapy is not warranted.
- Clinical depression, with symptoms including insomnia, loss of appetite and weight, feelings of helplessness, low self-esteem, self-blame, lack of drive, fatigue, indecisiveness, hopelessness, suicidal ideation, preoccupation with health problems either real or imagined. Psychological or psychiatric intervention is warranted. Pharmacotherapy as an adjunct.
- Emotional outbursts, anxiety, "bad nerves." Emotional lability may reflect changes in family dynamics. Counselling on stress reduction may be of benefit.
- Forgetfulness – this may be related to sleep deprivation as well as familial and social stressors. Counselling on stress reduction may be of benefit.

Depression may refer to a mood, symptom, or syndrome. Normal experience includes feelings of sadness or disappointment. When intensity, pervasiveness, and duration interfere with normal social or physiological functioning, then intervention is warranted. Traditional medical assumptions linking menopause and severe depression (involutional melancholia) historically originated in publications by eminent physicians offering analysis based upon opinion and sociocultural beliefs.[13,14] More recent studies show a decline in the prevalence of depression in this age group (45 to 64), including no worsening of depressive symptoms related to bereavement compared with other age groups.[15] A British prospective study underscores the importance of pre-existing health problems, stereotyped beliefs, and social factors in understanding symptoms of the climacteric.[16] The diagnostic DSM IV criteria for depression do not differ for the menopausal group. However, symptoms may pose a diagnostic challenge. This is resolved only by careful attention to the patient's presenting symptoms and observance of diagnostic criteria guidelines.

References

1. "Women and Mental Health in Canada: Strategies for Change," CMHA National Office 1987, 2160 Yonge Street, Toronto, ON M4S 2Z3.

2. de Souza M., "The Colours of Menopause," *Health Sharing* Winter 1990, 11(4): 14-17.

3. Flint M., "Cross-cultural factors that affect age of menopause," P.A. van Keep, R.B. Greenblatt, M. Albeaux-Fernet (eds): *Consensus in Menopausal Research. A Summary of International Opinion*, University Park Press, Baltimore, 1985: 73-85.

4. Erlik Y, I.V. Tataryn, D.R. Meldrum *et al.*, "Association of waking episodes with menopausal hot flushes," *JAMA* 1981, 245: 1741-1744.

5. Ballinger C.B., "Subjective sleep disturbance at menopause," *J. Psychosom. Res.* 1976, 20: 509-513.

6. Thomson J., I. Oswald, "Effect of oestrogen on the sleep, mood, and anxiety of menopausal women," *Br. Med. J.* 1977, 2: 1317-1319.

7. Hunter M., R. Battersby, M. Whitehead, "Relationships between psychological symptoms, somatic complaints and menopausal status," *Maturitas* 1986, 8: 217-228.

8. Glenn N.D., "Psychological well being in the post parental stage: some evidence from national surveys," *J. Marriage Family* 1975, 37: 105-110.

9. Greene J.G., D.J. Cooke, "Life stress and symptoms at the climacterium," *Br. J. Psychiat.* 1980, 136: 486-491.

10. Greene J.G., "Bereavement and social support at the climacteric," *Maturitas* 1983, 5: 115-124.

11. Koster A., "Change-of-life anticipations, attitudes, and experiences among middle-aged Danish women," *Health Care for Women International* 1991, 12: 1-13.

12. Planned Parenthood, "Facing the Change of Life - A Resource Kit on Menopause," Newfoundland, 1984, Session IV, 5-7.

13. Youngs D., "Some misconceptions concerning menopause," *Obstet. Gynecol.* 1990, 75: 881-883.

14. Weissman M.M., "The myth of involutional melancholia," *JAMA* 1979, 242: 742-744.

15. Myers J.K., M.M. Weissman, G.L. Tischler, "Six month prevalence of psychiatric disorders in three communities," *Arch. Gen. Psychiatry* 1984, 41: 959-967.

16. Hunter M., "The south-east England longitudinal study of the climacteric and post menopause," *Maturitas* 1992, 14: 117-126.

Sexual Transitions Associated with Menopause

Human sexuality is a life-long experiential process in which adaptation, innovation, and change characterize maturation. Sexuality includes emotional closeness or intimacy, sensual pleasure, physical and psychological responsiveness, and satisfaction. For women, the foundation of a positive experience of sexuality includes personal feelings of self-worth, a comfortable and communicative relationship characterized by mutual caring, and a (guilt-free) sense of fun and pleasure.

In 1975, the World Health Organization defined sexual health as "the integration of the somatic, emotional, intellectual and social aspects of sexual being, in ways that are positively enriching and that enhance personality, communication and love."[1]

The report cited three basic elements of sexual health:
- a capacity to enjoy and control sexual and reproductive behaviour in accordance with a social and personal ethic;
- freedom from fear, shame, guilt, false beliefs and other psychological factors inhibiting sexual response and impairing sexual relationship; and
- freedom from organic disorders, diseases and deficiencies that interfere with sexual and reproductive functions.

If these elements are present, the bodily changes of menopause and advancing years need not interfere with a sense of fulfilling sexuality.[2]

While sexual activity may continue throughout the aging process, there is a gradual change in sexual behaviour. Many etiological factors are involved. Discomfort and/or dyspareunia experienced by postmenopausal women are due to anatomical and physiological changes in the genital and extragenital tissue. The epidermis becomes thinner, the vagina becomes shorter, and elasticity is lost.[3] There is a loss of muscle tone and cervical secretion is decreased. An important factor in each phase of sexual response, from excitation to resolution, is an adequate circulation.[4] Decreased blood flow results in a gradual decrease in vulvar skin colour, and a decrease in clitoral and labial engorgement with sexual arousal. The ischemia is related to estrogen withdrawal and is improved by estrogen therapy.[5,6]

It appears that estrogen deficiency also affects peripheral nerve functioning. Resulting clinical symptoms include paresthesia and intolerance to touch.[7] Altered sensory perception can contribute to a loss of clitoral sensation and can affect the orgasmic response to sexual stimulation. There is a decrease in the size and volume of the orgasmic platform, in the orgasmic response to stimulation, and in the intensity of the pubococcygeal spasm and contractions of bladder and rectal muscles. There is also a necessity for increased amounts of stimulation to achieve maximum response. There is no change in the ability to achieve maximum response or in the ability to achieve single or multiple orgasms. These changes as described are age-related transitions occurring primarily in postmenopausal women. Women aged 40 to 55 are less likely to report experiencing symptoms (remembering that there is variance in hormonal status among women).

Kinsey *et al* [8] studied female sexuality throughout the life cycle, sampling a wide spectrum of the population. Decreased coital frequency and coitus leading to orgasm were found in women in the perimenopausal and postmenopausal age groups. Kinsey did not attribute this decline to the sexual capacity of women but rather to physiologic and psychologic changes in the male-female sexual relationship, primarily to a decline in male sexual functioning. Pfeiffer *et al* [9] also noted an age-related decline in sexual activity. The category "no interest in sex" was rated by 7% of the sample aged 40 to 55 years, increasing to 31% by those aged 56 to 60 years. The study content supported the Kinsey conclusion.

The availability of a responsive partner strongly determines sexual activity. At the same time as a woman experiences menopause, her male partner, now in his 50s, may experience changes in his sexual functioning, with delayed and/or partial erections (arteriosclerosis and reduced connective tissue elasticity), reduced fluid and force of ejaculation, prolonged plateau phase (sustained erection), more rapid detumescence after orgasm, and an increased refractory period before the next erection-ejaculation cycle.

An extensive survey of women one year postmenopause was conducted by Hällström.[10] The women studied showed a decline in sexual activity, with only 20% reporting weak or absent sexual interest at age 38 years. This number increased to 52% at age 54 years. This change was associated with a decline in the capacity for orgasm, an increase in dyspareunia, and a decrease in coital activity. Present understanding and treatment recommendation of female physiologic changes at menopause have led to a reduction in dyspareunia associated with urogenital atrophy and ischemic changes. The question remaining relates to the issue of sexual interest, arousal and pleasure in the perimenopause and postmenopause.

In a prospective study of middle-class North American women in the perimenopausal transition, clustered at ages 44 to 52, the majority evidenced changes in menstrual cycle length, bleeding patterns, hot flushes, night sweats, and emotional lability. Interestingly, there was a lack of a linear relationship between age and estradiol level marking the temporal individuality of each woman's cycle. Decreased coital frequency and atrophic changes in the lower genital tract were associated with very low (less than 35 pg/mL) serum estradiol concentration at any age. Regular weekly coital frequency appeared to maintain or to enhance vaginal lubrication, retard urogenital atrophy, and reduce the potential for dyspareunia. Estrogen decline had little, if any, effect on sexual desire, response, or satisfaction with sexual life in this group.[11]

In a Danish prospective population study, women who held cultural stereotypes of menopause as a period of decline (anticipated loss of sexuality and presumed increased ill health) were those to report a decrease in sexual drive and frequency in their fifties. As no correlation was found between hormonal status and decline in sexual desire or activity, it appears attitudes held concerning menopause markedly influence the woman's subjective experience of this stage of life.[12]

In women, atrophic urogenital changes may lead to problems of insertional dyspareunia, inadequate lubrication with arousal and orgasm, and post-coital bleeding. Over time, fear of coitus, vaginismus, and a consequent decline in sexual activity may result. Hot flushes, night sweats, and insomnia may adversely affect sexual desire. For these women, HRT, particularly estrogen, results in significant physiological improvement that may provide the context for sexual activity to proceed unimpaired.[13] The woman's self-perception of her own desirability may change her willingness to engage in sex and diminish sexual responsiveness. Couples who have long-established and satisfactory sex lives together may have sexual difficulties for the first time, while couples who have long-standing dysfunctions may find their problems exacerbated.[6] Sociocultural attitudes toward female sexuality after menopause traditionally have been negative. Recent data collected on women aged 39 to 65 years demonstrated that the majority of women who were optimistic in their attitude toward menopause had satisfactory sexual functioning.[14] Some women though, report sexual disinterest or decreased libido despite adequate HRT. Testosterone may be a hormone that is critically important to sexual desire in the surgically menopausal woman.

Physician counselling around issues of sexuality may initially occur with the woman individually. Ideally, her sexual partner should be invited to participate in educational, informative, and practical counselling sessions that both address and validate the physiological and psychological responses to the menopausal transition.

References

1. World Health Organization, "Education and Treatment in Human Sexuality: the Training of Health Professionals," *Technical Report Series* 572, WHO, Geneva, 1975: 6.

2. Renshaw D.C., "Sex, age and values," *J. Am. Geriat. Soc.* 1985, 33(9): 635-643.

3. Lang W.R., G.E. Aponte, "Gross and microscopic anatomy of the aged female reproductive organs," *Clin. Obstet. Gynecol.* 1967, 10: 454-465

4. Masters W, V. Johnson, "Human Sexual Inadequacy, Little Brown & Co., Boston, 1970.

5. Semmens J.P., G. Wagner, "Estrogen deprivation and vaginal function in postmenopausal women," *JAMA* 1982, 248: 445-448.

6. Sarrel L.J., P.M. Sarrel, "*Sexual Turning Points*," MacMillan, New York, 1984: 239-248.

7. Sarrel P.M., "Laser doppler measurement of peripheral blood flow," M. Notelovitz, P.A. van Keep (eds), *The Climacteric in Perspective*, MTP Press, Lancaster, 1986: 161-175.

8. Kinsey A.C., W.B. Pomeroy, C.E. Martin *et al*: *Sexual Behaviour in the Human Female*, WB Saunders, London, 1953: 734-736.

9. Pfeiffer E., A. Verwoerdt, G.C. Davis "Sexual behavior in middle life," *Am. J. Psychiat.* 1972, 128: 1262-1267.

10. Hällström T., "*Mental Disorder and Sexuality in the Climacteric. A Study in Psychiatric Epidemiology*," Esselte Studium, Goetbord, Sweden, 1973: 90-97.

11. Cutler W.B., C.R. Garcia, N. McCoy, "Perimenopausal sexuality," *Arch. Sex. Behav.* 1987, 16(3): 225-234.

12. Koster A., K. Garde, "Sexual desire and menopausal development. A prospective study of Danish women born in 1936," *Maturitas* 1993, 16: 49-60.

13. Walling M.A., B. Anderson, S.R. Johnson, "Hormonal replacement therapy for postmenopausal women. A review of sexual outcomes and related gynecological effects," *Arch. Sex. Behav.* 1990, 19: 119-137.

14. Bachman G.A., S.R. Leiblum, "Sexuality in sexagenarian women," *Maturitas* 1991; 13: 43-50.

Bone and Mineral Metabolism

Bone Remodelling

Continuous remodelling of bone appears to be necessary so that the strength of the skeleton and its physiological functions may be maintained. The bone remodelling cycle is defined as the ongoing cellular processes whereby old bone is continuously replaced by new bone throughout life. Bone can be considered to be made up of a number of bone multicellular units or bone remodelling units, the majority of which are quiescent or in a resting phase at any particular time. Activation of a new bone remodelling unit occurs about once every second in the normal adult skeleton and there are about 10 bone remodelling units in action at any one time. Activation of a remodelling unit is thought to be initiated by a chemical signal from osteoblasts, as a result of which osteoclasts are attracted to the bone surface and begin resorption. Osteoclast activity results in bone resorption and the formation of a pit or hole (lacuna) in the bone. This resorptive phase lasts 10 to 15 days, after which the lacuna is invaded by osteoblasts. The osteoblasts are thought to be attracted by chemical signals released from the bone matrix during its resorption by the osteoclast, principally insulin-like growth factor 1 (IGF-1).

In normal bone remodelling, the osteoblasts completely refill the lacuna excavated by the osteoclast. The total bone remodelling cycle lasts about four months in normal adults. Bone resorption is normally coupled to bone reformation in a steady state fashion and the result is a maintenance of bone mass. Throughout life there is a normal loss and replacement of bone. Until about age 35, bone formation predominates over bone loss. Both cortical and trabecular bone mass tend to increase to their peak in the mid-thirties, and be maintained until approximately the mid-forties in the absence of disease, inadequate diet, or certain hormonal disorders. At this age, osteoclastic activity begins to predominate and trabecular bone loss begins. Significant cortical loss does not begin until the fifties. The individual who has built up the greatest peak bone mass will be best protected from development of osteoporosis.

There is an accelerated but self-limiting period of bone loss during the five to ten years following menopause. Skeletal wasting with advancing age is more pronounced in white females than in white males, particularly those of slight build. Women eventually lose about 35% to 40% of their cortical bone mass and 55% to 60% of their trabecular bone. Men lose approximately two thirds of this amount. After 70 years of age, bone loss diminishes and the rate of loss in the closing years of life is approximately equal in both sexes.

Osteoporosis that occurs following menopause has been distinguished from the decline in bone mass associated with various disease states (secondary osteoporosis) and from that associated with aging (type II osteoporosis) by the designation type I osteoporosis. This condition is attributed largely to the decline in the level of estrogens and possibly progesterone. The mechanism by which estrogen protects against osteoporosis and fractures is not entirely clear, but is likely multifactorial. Estrogen deficiency increases the sensitivity of osteoclasts to parathormone and results in the excavation of deeper resorption lacunae. Estrogen deficiency may also impair osteoblast function since estrogen receptors have been demonstrated on osteoblasts.[1] Thirdly, there is some support in the literature for an effect of estrogen on vitamin D synthesis by the kidneys. Finally, estrogen deficiency leads to an increase in bone turnover as a result of more frequent activation of bone remodelling units. In this situation, since osteoblastic repair takes longer than osteoclastic resorption, the increase in activation frequency does not allow reformation to catch up to resorption and the result is a decrease in bone mass.

The mechanism of the increased activation of bone remodelling units in the presence of estrogen deficiency and the protective effect of estrogen replacement to slow down bone turnover again is unclear, but may be modulated by cytokines such as interleukin-1 (IL-1) or interleukin-6 (IL-6). There is indirect evidence to support this hypothesis since activated monocytes produce IL-1 and IL-1 may activate bone remodelling units. Menopause, or estrogen deficiency from any cause, is associated with increased IL-1 production by bone associated mono-cytes. Pacifici *et al.*[2] demonstrated that estrogen replacement therapy is associa-ted with decreased IL-1 production and this may be the mechanism through which activation of bone remodelling units is decreased in the presence of HRT.

Progesterone production from the ovaries may also play a significant role in maintenance of bone mass on premenopausal women. Ericksen *et al.*[1] demonstrated the presence of progesterone receptors on osteoblastic cells and it is possible that progesterone or progestins will stimulate osteoblastic bone formation.[3] Recently, Prior *et al.*[4] in Vancouver suggested that progesterone deficiency related to anovulatory cycles or even subtle progesterone deficiency, such as seen with luteal phase defects, could result in a significant reduction in bone mass in premenopausal women.[4] This observation needs to be confirmed but, if correct, indicates that progesterone may be important in the prevention of osteoporosis.

Risk Factors for Osteoporosis

Established risk factors for osteoporosis include premature menopause, menopause, a positive family history, Caucasian or Oriental race, small stature, low body weight, low calcium intake, physical inactivity or levels of activity sufficiently high to cause oligomenorrhea or amenorrhea, nulliparity, smoking, alcohol abuse, excessive caffeine intake, excessive protein intake, excessive intake of vitamins A or D, eating disorders, gastric or small bowel resection, a history of hyperthyroidism, and the use of adrenal corticosteroids, anticonvulsants, heparin and possibly other types of anticoagulants, cyclosporin, azathioprine and methotrexate.

Measurement of Bone Mass

Plain radiographs are of limited value for this purpose. However, bone mineral density (BMD) is highly correlated with bone strength [5] and ultimately with the risk of fracture.[6] BMD can be measured by single or dual photon absorptiometry by CT scan and, more recently, by dual x-ray absorptiometry (DEXA).

References

1. Eriksen E.F., D.S. Colvard, N.J. Berg *et al.*, "Evidence of estrogen-receptors in normal human osteoblast-like cells," *Science* 1988, 241: 84-86.

2. Pacifici R., C. Brown, E. Puscheck *et al.*, "Effect of surgical menopause and estrogen replacement on cytokine release from human blood mononuclear cells," *Proc. Natl. Acad. Sci. USA* 1991, 88: 5134-5138.

3. Christiansen C., L. Nilas, B.J. Riis *et al.*, "Uncoupling of bone formation and resorption by combined oestrogen and progestagen therapy in postmenopausal osteoporosis," *Lancet* 1985, ii: 800-801.

4. Prior J.C., Y.M. Vigna, M.T. Schechter *et al*, "Spinal bone loss and ovulatory disturbances," *N. Engl. J. Med.* 1990, 323: 1221-1227.

5. Mazess R.B., "On aging bone loss," *Clin. Orthop.* 1982, 165: 239-252.

6. Melton L.J., H.W. Wahner, L.S. Richelson *et al.*, "Osteoporosis and the risk of hip fracture," *Am. J. Epidemiol.* 1986, 124: 254-261.

Cardiovascular System Changes

Cardiovascular disease increases with age. Before menopause, women have a relatively lower overall risk of cardiovascular disease than their male counterparts. This selective benefit decreases after surgical or natural menopause but is partially restored by estrogen replacement. Cardiovascular disease is the major cause of mortality in women. The positive role of HRT is discussed in more detail later in this document.

The Framingham Study and many others show that in Western society, women have a consistently lower rate of ischemic heart disease than men. The rate of ischemic heart disease in women is relatively constant up to the age of 40. After 40 the rate increases and runs parallel, but at a lower overall rate to the age-matched male population.[1] The relative differences in male-female ischemic heart disease rates vary greatly between different geographic populations, although the direction of effect is constant. Besides being an important source of morbidity, cardiovascular disease is the main cause of death in women in the 50 to 80 age group.[2] Recent mortality statistics in the United States indicate that the lifetime risk of cardiovascular death in women approaches 60%. This is 10 times the risk of any other disease, including breast cancer. Before menopause, approximately the same number of women die from myocardial infarction as from breast cancer. After menopause, the rate of death from myocardial infarction far exceeds the rate from breast cancer.[3] Cardiovascular disease accounts for more deaths of women in the United States than do all forms of cancer combined.

The suggestion has been made, on the basis of beneficial cholesterol and lipoprotein profiles with exogenous estrogen, that endogenous estrogen protects against the development of cardiovascular disease by altering lipid and lipoprotein metabolism favourably. An extrapolation of these observations is that exogenous estrogen administration to postmenopausal women may delay the onset of atherosclerosis. There also may be evidence for direct protective effects of estrogen against cardiovascular disease at the level of the blood vessel wall and these data will be discussed later in the section Hormone Replacement Therapy: Pharmacology of Estrogen and Progestine Replacement (Chapter 5).

References

1. Castelli W.P., "Epidemiology of coronary heart disease: the Framingham Study. *Am. J. Med.* 1984, 76(2A): 4-12.

2. National Center for Health Statistics, "Vital Statistics of the United States 1981, Mortality Part A 1981," Hyattville, MD, 1986.

3. Grimes D.A., "Prevention of cardiovascular disease in women: role of the obstetrician-gynecologist," *Am. J. Obstet. Gynecol.* 1988, 158(suppl): 1662-1668.

5. Management of the Patient

Counselling

Menopause is not a disease state, but a transition in life which is passed by every normal woman. It is a physiologic change as a result of cessation of ovarian function, with a gradual reduction in ovarian hormones, and increasing evidence of estrogen deprivation in target tissues. It is a period of life that is misunderstood, shadowed in myth, and often feared by women and their families.

Many women confuse menopause, the last occurrence of physiological bleeding (menstruation), with the climacteric, which is the change from reproductive to non-reproductive status. In order that women may come to terms with these changes, positive and sensitive counselling is essential. The counselling must present information in such a way that the woman understands the physiological changes that are taking place in her body and can discuss her concerns without embarrassment. In an ideal situation, counselling in the medical setting should begin during a health maintenance visit, often called the well woman visit at the time of the Pap smear, when the woman is in her thirties, and should be followed by further counselling when the woman is perimenopausal (in her forties), menopausal (in her fifties), and postmenopausal (in her sixties). Special consideration and advice is necessary for the woman who has had a medically or surgically induced menopause.

Counselling in the thirties

The premenopausal visit may be the most strategic concerned with counselling on menopause. At this visit, menopause can be defined and its physiology explained. Questions can be addressed, and expectations and myths should be explored. Negative attitudes to menopause are more prevalent in younger women than in perimenopausal or postmenopausal women; this is the time to redress misinformation.[1]

All women will develop osteoporosis to some degree. The premenopausal visit should focus on the woman's ability to delay osteoporosis by developing good health habits of proper diet and exercise. Bone mass starts to decrease in the mid-thirties. It is important for women to reach their optimal peak bone mass before bone loss begins, and to maintain their bone mass as much as possible. There are several well-documented risk factors for osteoporosis, including Caucasian race, a positive family history, small body build, and nulliparity. Three important risk factors can be minimized by the woman herself: inadequate dietary calcium intake, insufficient weight-bearing exercise, and excessive alcohol intake. Heavy use of tobacco or caffeine; diets high in protein, sodium, or phosphate; and a low intake of vitamin D also increase the risk. Bone formation is dependent upon both adequate calcium intake and exercise, as the calcium uptake by bone increases in proportion to the mechanical stress placed on bone during exercise.[2]

Exercise is known to have a positive effect on bone density. Bone growth is stimulated by the mechanical load of exercise, muscular activity, and gravity. For this reason, the exercise must be weightbearing; horizontal exercise is not beneficial. The duration and frequency of exercise required to protect against postmenopausal osteoporosis is yet to be determined accurately.[3]

Calcium intake from diet and supplements, in this age group, should total 1000 to 1500 mg per day.[4] Unfortunately, many adults stop drinking milk when teenagers; bones continue to grow until age 35. The diet should be reviewed and information provided on calcium requirements. An intake of four cups of milk (300 mg calcium per 8 oz. serving) per day or its equivalent in other dairy products and foods is recommended. If the dietary intake is insufficient, calcium supplements should be prescribed. Attention needs to be paid to the amount of elemental calcium rather than calcium salt in commercial supplements. As for any medication, patient compliance can be encouraged by considering cost, acceptability, and convenience. Calcium excretion is enhanced by alcohol, caffeine, and smoking. Moderation should be advised and smoking discouraged.

Women should eat a diet rich in whole grains, fruit, and low fat dairy products. Very thin women should try to gain some weight because they seem to have less natural estrogen after menopause (adipose tissue can produce estrone) and may have an increased risk for the development of osteoporosis.

Counselling in the forties

The perimenopausal visit(s) should focus on the changes that may be expected from aging and estrogen deprivation. The majority of women do not suffer severe symptoms from estrogen deficiency, but unfortunately there is a growing belief that estrogen will cure all ills. Realistic expectations should be discussed. As a general rule, estrogen is not indicated for this age group, unless a deficiency is identified by appropriate laboratory investigations. Menstrual irregularities often precede menopause; normal and abnormal patterns should be discussed, always emphasizing the normal physiological changes.

These sessions provide an opportunity to explore the area of sexual activity. It offers the woman a chance to ask questions and raise concerns she may have about sexual function later in life. After menopause has been explained to her, specific information should be given on clinical entities that result from estrogen deficiency, such as hot flushes, genitourinary atrophy, osteoporosis, and cardiovascular disease.

Special attention must be given to the woman who has had a surgical menopause. The manifestations of estrogen deficiency are more severe and of more abrupt onset for surgical than for natural menopause, and estrogen replacement is more important in the younger woman, to prevent the morbidity and mortality of osteoporosis and cardiovascular disease over an extended postmenopausal lifetime. Counselling and education may be required as the woman is experiencing menopause at an earlier age than her peers.

Women who have had a hysterectomy without a bilateral oophorectomy will not have menstrual irregularities to prompt a visit to the doctor. They need to be followed carefully with enquiries about menopausal symptoms and screening for estrogen deficiency.

Menopausal flushes

The section on Hot Flushes (Chapter 4) outlines the physiology of the event and the role of estrogen. However, symptomatic women need to be offered simple solutions in order to keep themselves comfortable. Cool clothes, made of cotton material with an open neck, are helpful. If the clothing is put on in layers, the top layer can be more easily removed discretely if necessary. At night, a cool shower before retiring, cotton sheets, and a pitcher of ice water at the bedside are helpful. Precipitating factors for hot flushes include caffeine, alcohol, and spicy foods.

Osteoporosis

Ideally, osteoporosis will have been discussed at a premenopausal visit in the thirties. Preventive measures that have already been instituted with respect to calcium intake, exercise, and dietary habits should be reviewed and reinforced. If this is the first opportunity to discuss osteoporosis, a more thorough explanation and preventive regimen will be required, as outlined earlier.

Genitourinary atrophy

Less estrogen is required to maintain the endometrium than the vaginal and urethral mucosa. Symptoms of genitourinary atrophy may therefore occur before cessation of the menses.[5] The main symptoms are those of urethritis (dysuria, frequency, urgency, and nocturia with a sterile urine culture) and dyspareunia.

Hormone replacement therapy (HRT) will relieve the symptoms most effectively. General methods of relief should be advised and may consist of adequate fluid intake, Kegel exercises, and urinary analgesics such as phenazopyridine. Urethral dilatation may be necessary. For friable vulvar tissue, surgical water-soluble jelly, lanolin, and mineral oil are suitable lubricants for intercourse; cosmetic creams are not. Soaps may be irritating or drying, particularly if they contain detergent, and they should not be used.

Sexuality

The prevalent myth that the loss of ovarian function means the end of sexuality should be dispelled. Neither age nor estrogen deprivation will cause sexual dysfunction in a healthy aging person who has continued to be sexually active. Vaginal dryness and associated atrophic changes in the mucous membrane, decreased desire, and diminished response are the commonest sexual complaints of the menopausal woman. While HRT can be beneficial in the management of local changes in the genitourinary tract and therefore indirectly in the enjoyment of sex, it is not certain that estrogen has any direct effect on desire and response. It is ideal, therefore, that any treatment be accompanied by sex counselling which includes the partner, and should provide information and reassurance to the couple about sexuality in the older man and woman. It may be necessary to emphasize that sexual relations are not only normal at menopause, but healthy, and help to maintain the genitourinary tissues. However, if there has been an interruption of sexual activity as a result of separation or illness, there may be some discomfort on resumption of activity.

It is important to review the possible causes of sexual dysfunction, and to differentiate between physiological genitourinary atrophy and loss of libido due to an unsatisfactory sexual relationship or concomitant depression.

Counselling in the fifties

In the years following cessation of menstruation, bothersome menopausal symptoms appear. There is tremendous individual variation in the severity of these symptoms. It is estimated that only 25% of women will have menopausal symptoms severe enough to seek treatment. The symptoms of genitourinary atrophy and osteoporosis can remain silent for five to ten years. The decision to use estrogen should not be based solely on the presence of symptoms because many more women will benefit from the preventive use of HRT.[6]

Counselling of the menopausal woman must review the advantages and disadvantages and alternatives to HRT, so that the woman can make an informed choice about her health care. Diet and exercise again should be discussed. Calcium intake is recommended as 1500 mg per day. Counselling regarding sexuality is concerned with the same issues outlined previously. The woman may present with clearly defined symptoms or issues at this stage. The office visit should also include a complete physical examination in order to establish baselines for the postmenopausal period.

Screening for cancer

- Breast Cancer

The Canadian Workshop Group on Mammography recommended a clinical breast examination (CBE) annually by a trained health professional as part of a complete breast assessment in women over the age of 40 years.[7] The breasts should be examined both in the sitting and recumbent positions and include the regional lymphatics; anterior, cervical supraclavicular, and axillary compartments. The recumbent position affords the best access to the axillary tail. Breast cancer will be detectable by CBE when mammography is negative in approximately 13% of women aged 40 to 49 years and in 6% of women over the age of 50 years.

Breast self-examination (BSE) has generated considerable controversy among physicians as it is difficult to standardize and evaluate. Most cancers are initially felt by women themselves. Women trained in BSE can detect smaller tumours. By the age of 40, women should be practising BSE on a regular basis. Women in their thirties, and women of all ages with a history of breast cancer in a first degree relative, should be taught BSE.[8,9]

For the early detection of breast cancer, screening of asymptomatic women between the ages of 50 and 69 years was recommended by the Canadian Workshop Group on Mammography. An initial mammogram at age 50, followed by one every second year, was proposed. The American Cancer Society endorses early screening beginning at age 40.[10]

All consensus groups now clearly recommend screening mammography for asymptomatic women over 50 years of age although there continues to be controversy over the cost-effectiveness of screening women under 50 and over 70 years of age. These groups agree that symptomatic women, irrespective of age, need diagnostic mammography. Moreover, women with a strong family history of breast cancer, particularly in a sister or mother who developed the disease before menopause, should commence mammography five to ten years before the youngest case of breast cancer in the family. In addition, annual or biannual CBE is indicated at age 30 years for this population.

● Cancer of the Cervix

The report from the National Workshop on Screening for Cancer of the Cervix suggested an initial Pap smear at age 18 years, followed by a second smear one year later.[11] After two satisfactory smears showing no significant epithelial abnormality, women should be screened every three years to the age of 69 years. This is based upon the availability of a standard Pap smear registry. As standardization of the provincial pathology registries has not yet been achieved, individual provinces are still making recommendations based upon the exigencies of the regions.

If abnormalities are detected by a Pap smear, the schedule for repeat examinations should be dictated by the requirements of surveillance, diagnosis, treatment, and follow-up. The presence of cervical intraepithelial neoplasia (CIN) Grade I to III or actual malignancy requires referral for colposcopic examination.

Counselling in the sixties

Many women do not realize that an annual postmenopausal health check-up is as important as in the premenopausal years, and this must be emphasized to the patient. Postmenopausal counselling should review menopausal symptoms and concerns. The role of exercise and diet in slowing the development of osteoporosis should be reinforced. Symptoms that are the result of estrogen deficiency (hot flushes, discomfort as a result of genitourinary atrophy) should be discussed.

If the woman is taking HRT, its use should be reviewed. It is advised at this time to enquire about any abnormal vaginal bleeding and to arrange for its investigation.

During this visit, it is also wise to begin discussions on retirement planning. Many communities have excellent resources, with self-help groups for medical and social problems (such as loneliness). Women should be given full information on the facilities that are available. The introduction of counselling sessions on menopause early in a woman's life should minimize the apprehension associated with menopause, decrease her risk of osteoporosis, and optimize her health. Such counselling should be scheduled annually. Physicians should strive to incorporate menopausal counselling into their overall approach to health maintenance visits.

References

1. Greene J.G., "*Social and Psychological Origins of the Climacteric Syndrome*," Gower Publishing Ltd., Aldershot, Hants, England, 1984.

2. Martin A.D., C.S. Houston, "Osteoporosis, calcium and physical activity," *Can. Med. Assoc. J.* 1987, 136: 587-593.

3. Smith E.L. Jr, P.E. Smith, C.J. Ensign *et al.*, "Bone involution decreases in exercising middle-aged women," *Calcif. Tissue Int.* 1984, 36(suppl 1): S129-S138.

4. Consensus Conference, "Osteoporosis," *JAMA* 1984, 252: 799-802.

5. Semmens J.P., E.C. Semmens, "Sexual function and menopause," *Clin. Obstet. Gynecol.* 1984, 27: 717-723.

6. Utian W.H., "Current status of menopause and post-menopausal estrogen therapy," *Obstet. Gynecol. Surv.* 1977, 32: 193-204.

7. Workshop report, "Reducing deaths from breast cancer in Canada," *Can. Med. Assoc. J.* 1989, 141: 199-201.

8. Chart P.L., G.A. Taylor, "Ensuring detection of breast cancer," *Can. J. Diagn.* 1991, 7: 54-73.

9. Yaffe M., "Ontario Breast Screening Program position paper," 1990.

10. Buring J.E., C.H. Hennekens, R.J. Lipnick *et al.*, "A prospective study of postmenopausal hormone use and risk of cancer in US women," *Am. J. Epidemiol.* 1987, 125(6): 939-946.

11. Miller A.B., G. Anderson, J. Brisson *et al.*, "Report of a national workshop on screening for cancer of the cervix," *Can. Med. Assoc. J.* 1991, 145: 1301-1325.

Contraception in Perimenopausal Patients

In Canada, about half of perimenopausal women are not at risk of pregnancy because one or both partners has elected to undergo sterilization. According to Fédération CECOS,[1] the fecundity rate decreases with advancing age, especially over 45. However, as a rule, any woman who is menstruating regularly must be regarded as ovulating regularly.

In pregnancies occurring in the perimenopause, smoking, obesity, hypertension, cardiovascular changes, and diabetes are complicating factors. In addition, risks for the fetus are increased in relation to the greater frequency of chromosomal abnormalities, such as autosomal trisomies and sex chromosome abnormalities (XXY and XXX), spontaneous abortion, and perinatal mortality.[2]

Spontaneous abortions occur three times more often in the 40- to 44-year-old age group and five times more in those 45 years or over, compared to those in younger women. Consequently, one pregnancy out of three will end in a spontaneous abortion between ages 40 to 44 and one pregnancy out of two after age 45.[3]

At age 35, the risk of having a live born infant with a significant chromosomal abnormality is approximately 1 in 200. This risk rises to approximately 1 in 20 at age 45. Specific rates for chromosomal abnormalities in relation to maternal age have been approximately 30% higher in prenatal diagnostic studies than in live births, which is partly due to the increased spontaneous abortion rates associated with trisomies (13, 18, 21) and Turner's syndrome (45, X).[4]

Increased maternal and fetal morbidity and mortality are common and should be discussed with perimenopausal patients who are not using contraceptives. The choice of a contraceptive method in this age group should be made after a thorough discussion of difficulties associated with contraceptive use, such as increased cardiovascular risk with oral contraceptives or uncertainty with ovulation time related to menstrual cycle length (rhythm method). In the case of irregular and anovulatory cycles that are often observed in the perimenopausal years, contraceptive efficacy may be reduced by inconsistent use. However, in the general discussion that precedes the selection of a method, the patient should be told that an IUD, spermicide, condom, or diaphragm, because of her decreasing fertility rate and lowered incidence of pelvic infection, may represent a more proper choice and an alternative to surgical sterilization.

Contraceptive Methods

IUDs

Recently, Kozuh-Novak and Andolsek[5] have stated that the IUD is one of the most appropriate contraceptive methods for women over age 40. There are fewer infections, removals, and side effects in older women. Consequently, IUDs in this age group have better efficacy, are better tolerated, and are associated with less pelvic infection. Gyne-T 380® and Nova T® need not be removed for seven years, especially at this age because of the decrease in fertility rate and long duration of effectiveness.[6,7]

Natural (rhythm) methods
(Billings, basal body temperature, symptothermic)

Because of a frequent shortening of the length of the follicular phase after the age of 40, and especially after 45,[8] these natural contraceptive methods may have reduced efficacy unless combined with chemical or barrier methods.

Chemical and barrier methods

Diaphragms, condoms, sponges, and spermicides are efficacious and well accepted in this period of life and they have lower morbidity and mortality rates than any other means of contraception.[9]

Hormonal contraception

Data continue to accumulate regarding the safety of low-dose oral contraceptive (OC) use among women over the age of 35 who have no contraindications to OC use and are otherwise in good health. Smoking remains the major risk factor for women over the age of 35. Women who smoke should not use oral contraceptives beyond the age of 35 years. Current scientific opinion reflects that the relative safety of the low-dose OCs, combined with the well-established non-contraceptive benefits of these pills for women beyond the age of 35 who do not smoke and are in otherwise good health outweighs the potential risks which may occur due to OC use.[10] An increased risk of cardiovascular disease that may be attributed to OC use remains a possibility in this population. The risk, however, may be less than those associated with pregnancy and alternative surgical and medical procedures that may be needed should pregnancy occur. The lowest possible dose formulation compatible with a high level of efficacy, a low incidence of side effects, and good cycle control should be employed.

Injectable and implantable progestin contraceptives

These preparations are an alternative to oral contraceptives. They are effective, but may increase body weight, and cause amenorrhea and menstrual irregularities. However, there is no significant change in lipid metabolism, nor in the incidence of thromboembolic or cardiovascular disease.[11,12] There also may be a beneficial effect in the prevention of endometrial carcinoma.

Sterilization

Although this method is almost 100% effective, it carries a surgical risk and does not prevent the increasing menstrual problems that are often observed in this age group. The short period of usefulness of sterilization after the age of 45 should be weighed against the surgical risk of the method.

At what age may contraception be discontinued?

Whenever amenorrhea of six months' duration is observed in association with an increase in serum follicle stimulating harmone (FSH) over 40 IU/L, the chance of the patient becoming pregnant is less than 1/100 and contraception may reasonably be stopped.

References

1.   Fédération CECOS, D. Schwartz, M.J. Mayaux, "Female fecundity as a function of age. results of artificial insemination in 2193 nulliparous women with azoospermic husbands," *N. Engl. J. Med.* 1982, 306: 404-406.

2.   Schreinemachers D.M., P.K. Cross, E.B. Hook, "Rates of trisomies 21, 18, 13 and other chromosome abnormalities in about 20,000 prenatal studies compared with estimated rates in live births," *Hum. Genet.* 1982, 61: 318-324.

3.   Warburton D., "Outcome of cases of de novo structural rearrangements diagnosed at amniocentesis," *Prenat. Diagn.* 1984, 4(spec. no.): 69-80.

4.   Hook E.B., "Chromosome abnormalities and spontaneous fetal death following amniocentesis: further data and associations with maternal age," *Am. J. Hum. Genet.* 1983, 35: 110-116.

5.   Kozuh-Novak M., L. Andolsek, "IUD use after 40 years of age," *Adv. Contracep.* 1988, 4: 85-94.

6.   Sivin I, J. Stern, E. CoutinHo *et al.*, "Prolonged intrauterine contraception: a seven-year randomized study of Levonorgestrel 20 mcg/day and the Copper T 380 Ag IUDs," *Contraception* 1991, 44: 473-480.

7.   Mishell D.R. Jr, "Editor's comments," *Yearbook of Obstetrics and Gynecology* 1993: 45.

8.   M. Vessey, Lawless M, Yeates D., "Efficacy of different contraceptive methods," *Lancet* 1982, i: 841-842.

9.   Tietze C., S. Lewit, "Life risks associated with reversible methods of fertility regulation," *Int. J. Gynaecol. Obstet.* 1978-1979, 16: 456-459.

10.   Godsland I.F., D. Crook, V. Wynn, "Clinical and metabolic considerations of long-term oral contraceptive use," *Am. J. Obstet. Gynecol.* 1992, 166: 1955-1963.

11.   Singh K., O.A.C. Viegas, D.F.M. Loke, S.S. Ratnam, "Effect of Norplant implants on liver, lipid and carbohydrate metabolism," *Contraception* 1992, 45: 141-153.

12.   Sivin I., J. Stern, S. Diaz *et al.*, "Rates and outcomes of planned pregnancy after use of Norplant capsules, Norplant II Rods, or Levonorgestrel-Releasing or Copper TCU 380 Ag Intrauterine contraceptive devices," *Am. J. Obstet. Gynecol.* 1992, 166: 1208-1213.

Hormone Replacement Therapy: Pharmacology of Estrogen and Progestin Replacement

Introduction

An estrogen is a steroid hormone that acts through a specific binding protein (receptor) to stimulate growth of Müllerian system-derived tissue and of female secondary sexual characteristics. Estrogen action may also influence "non-reproductive" tissues either directly through receptor mediation (e.g., brain, osteoblasts) or indirectly, through other hormonal systems (e.g., calcium metabolism). Estrogen acts as an inducer of both estrogen and progesterone receptors to enhance the efficacy of both steroids in target tissues.[1,2] A progestin is any analogue of progesterone that exerts biologic effects through specific progesterone receptors usually induced by, and found in the same tissues as, estrogen receptors. Progestins are also able to interfere with the binding sites of other hormones, consequently exhibiting both antiestrogenic [2,3] and, depending on the type of progestin, either androgenic or antiandrogenic actions.

Mechanism of Action of Estrogen and Progestin

Steroid hormones initiate their biologic activity through binding to intracellular receptor proteins that appear to be relatively (but not exclusively) specific for individual hormones. Classically, steroid receptors were thought to be located in the cytoplasm, and once bound by a steroid hormone, the hormone-receptor complex was translocated to the nucleus to interact with DNA.[4] More recent evidence, from studies [5,6] that avoided cellular disruption and used highly specific monoclonal antibodies against receptor protein, demonstrated that unoccupied steroid receptors are present mainly in the nucleus and not in cytoplasm. It is likely that steroid hormones, which are lipid soluble, diffuse into the nucleus where they bind to receptors that interact with DNA. This effect results in synthesis of messenger RNA (mRNA), which is transported out of the nucleus to cytoplasmic ribosomes. Activated by mRNA, the ribosomes manufacture proteins unique to the specific target cell.

Metabolism of Estrogens and Progestins

The biologic activity of estradiol is related to the free steroid which comprises 2% to 3% of circulating estradiol.[7] The rest of circulating estradiol is bound to plasma proteins such as sex hormone binding globulin (SHBG) (38%) and albumin (60%). Estradiol is metabolized by 17β-hydroxysteroid dehydrogenase to the less biologically active hormone, estrone.[8] Estrone is further metabolized to estriol by 16-hydroxylation[9] and to catecholestrogens by 2-hydroxylation.[10] Estradiol metabolites are conjugated in the liver to glucuronides and sulphates for excretion in the urine or bile.

Progesterone is bound to albumin and to a lesser degree to cortisol-binding globulin (CBG) in the circulation resulting in rapid clearance from blood.[11] Progesterone is metabolized to 20α-dihydroprogesterone,[11] which has weak progestational activity, and both progesterones are further metabolized to pregnanediol. Pregnanediol is conjugated to glucuronide and excreted in the urine.

Estrogens

Categorization of estrogens

Estrogens can be categorized by biochemical make-up (steroidal versus nonsteroidal) or origin (natural versus synthetic), as demonstrated in Table 2.

Table 2:
Categorization of estrogens

A. Natural Steroidal Estrogens
      Estradiol
      Estrone and estrone sulphate
      Estriol
      Conjugated estrogens
      Equine estrogens

B. Synthetic Steroidal Estrogens
      Esters of estradiol
      17α-ethinyl estrogens

C. Nonsteroidal Estrogens
      Diethylstilbestrol
      Dienestrol
      Chlorotrianisene

Estrogen pharmacology

A. Natural steroidal estrogens

Estradiol: When given orally, estradiol is poorly absorbed, except for a micronized preparation in which estradiol crystals are reduced in size to one to three microns. Most of orally administered micronized estradiol is converted in the gut to estrone sulphate[12] resulting in a pronounced estrone/estradiol ratio in the circulation. Intranasal[13] and sublingual[14] administration also result in marked serum increases in estrone sulphate levels. However, micronized estradiol is rapidly absorbed through the vaginal mucosa without being metabolized, thus resulting in a predominant increase in serum estradiol concentrations.[13] Recently, a transdermal delivery system has been developed for estradiol administration that bypasses the portal circulation and results in absorption of estradiol without major interconversion to estrone.[15] This method of delivery may be of value in patients in whom there is a history of poor gastrointestinal absorption or tolerance of oral estrogen preparations or in whom the first pass effect through the liver should be avoided.

Estrone and estrone sulphate: Like estradiol, estrone given orally is poorly absorbed and to be clinically useful, estrone sulphate is stabilized with piperazine. Piperazine estrone sulphate administration results in predominant serum concentrations of estrone sulphate with a serum estrone-estradiol ratio not unlike that seen with oral estradiol administration.[16]

Conjugated equine estrogens: The most commonly prescribed oral estrogen is a combination of conjugated equine estrogens (70% estrone sulphate, 20% equilin sulphate and equilenin sulphate, and 10% others). The estrone sulphates and the equine estrogens are absorbed orally with the latter steroids being relatively potent because of resistance to metabolism in the human. The equine estrogens are likely the reason why this preparation is two to three times more active at hepatic enzyme induction and promotion of globulin formation than preparations containing estrogens (estrone sulphate, estradiol) that occur naturally in the human.[17,18]

B.   Synthetic steroidal estrogens

Estrogen esters: Estradiol esters may be formed that are administered as solutions in oil or as aqueous suspensions intramuscularly. Examples are estradiol cypionate and estradiol valerate. When given I.M., these forms of estrogen have a gradual onset of action of relatively long duration. Some esters such as estradiol benzoate and valerate are also active orally.

17α-ethinyl estradiol: These estrogen preparations include ethinyl estradiol and mestranol, the estrogen components of oral contraceptives. The addition of the ethinyl group at the 17 position makes these estrogens orally active and retards metabolism, resulting in an increase in potency.[19] These estrogens are the most potent for clinical use but because of their relatively high estrogenic activity, these dosage formulations are usually not used for menopausal replacement.

C.   Nonsteroidal estrogens

Diethylstilbestrol is the most important estrogen of this group and was widely used in the 1940s and 1950s. Recent observations of teratogenic effects in offspring of women given this hormone during pregnancy[20] have virtually curtailed its use. These estrogens are not used at the present time for estrogen replacement therapy.

Progestins

Categorization of progestins

Progestins can be categorized as natural or synthetic and the synthetics can be further classified as C21 or C18 (19-nortestosterone) derivatives (Table 3).

Table 3:
Categorization of progestins

A.   Natural
    Progesterone

B.   Synthetic
    C21 derivatives
        Medroxyprogesterone acetate
        Cyproterone acetate
    C18 (19-nortestosterone) derivatives
        Norethindrone
        Levonorgestrel
        Desogestrel
        Gestodene
        Norgestimate

Progestin pharmacology

A.   Natural Progestins

Progesterone: Natural progesterone is poorly absorbed orally but can be micronized similar to estradiol to enhance oral efficacy. Micronized progesterone (200 mg) administered daily results in stable plasma progesterone levels in the range of 8 ng/mL.[21] At this physiologic dose, natural progesterone has been shown to have mild tranquillizing effects[22] and to antagonize the effect of estrogen replacement on the endometrium.[23]

B.   Synthetic Progestins

C21 derivatives:
- Medroxyprogesterone acetate

This progestin is well absorbed orally and is presently the most commonly used preparation to antagonize the endometrial proliferative effects of estrogen replacement therapy. At a dose of 5 mg daily, medroxyprogesterone acetate will induce biochemical and histological changes in the endometrium of estrogen-treated women equivalent to those seen in the secretory phase of the menstrual cycle.[23] At this dosage, medroxyprogesterone acetate has no demonstrable adverse effects on low density lipoprotein (LDL)- or high density lipoprotein (HDL)-cholesterol metabolism.[24]

- Cyproterone acetate

Cyproterone acetate has potent progestational activity when administered orally but is also one of the most potent antiandrogens presently available. It has been studied for the treatment of hirsutism,[25] and because of its antagonism of androgenic activity it may have a beneficial effect on lipid metabolism when combined with estrogen replacement.

C18 (19-nortestosterone) derivatives:
These potent progestins, found in oral contraceptives, are active at both progesterone and androgen receptors. At high-doses (10 mg of norethindrone, 0.5 mg levonorgestrel), these progestins have been shown to have a significant detrimental effect on lipid metabolism by decreasing the plasma concentration of HDL-C[24], likely because of their androgenic activity. The daily dose of each progestin capable of inducing endometrial secretory changes similar to those in the luteal phase of the menstrual cycle is 0.35 mg and 0.075 mg, respectively.[23] It is likely that no adverse effect on HDL-C occurs at these doses.

The new third generation progestins such as desogestrel, gestodene, and norgestimate are also 19-nortestosterone derivatives similar to norgestrel. However, in contrast to norethindrone and norgestrel, they have relatively low affinity for androgen receptors while retaining potent progestational activity. As a result, these progestins should have little negative effect on lipoprotein metabolism and may be ideal for use in HRT.

Pharmacodynamics of Estrogen and Progestin

Estrogen

In Canada, hormone replacement consists of the administration of estrogens such as conjugated estrogen, piperazine estrone sulphate, micronized estradiol, or estradiol with a transdermal therapeutic system, at a dose sufficient to approximate circulating levels of estrone and estradiol in the follicular phase of the menstrual cycle. Estrogen concentrations in premenopausal women in the early follicular phase, and in postmenopausal women, before and after 25 days' treatment with various doses of natural estrogens administered orally, are shown in Table 4.

Table 4:

Mean (± SEM) serum estradiol, estrone, and free estradiol in pg/mL in premenopausal (early follicular phase) and postmenopausal women before and after oral estrogen therapy

	Estradiol	Free Estradiol	Estrone
Premenopausal (follicular)	63 ± 15	17 ± 2	56 ± 5
Postmenopausal (untreated control)	10 ± 1	4 ± 1	37 ± 4
Conjugated Estrogen			
0.3 mg	19 ± 2	4 ± 1	76 ± 14
0.625 mg	39 ± 11	11 ± 4	153 ± 31
Estrone Sulphate			
0.6 mg	34 ± 7	12 ± 2	125 ± 25
1.2 mg	42 ± 7	11 ± 2	285 ± 52
Micronized Estradiol			
1.0 mg	30 ± 7	9 ± 2	266 ± 64

Adapted from Lobo R. *et al.*[26]

In studies on postmenopausal women using a transdermal system delivering 0.025, 0.05, or 0.1 mg of exogenous estradiol-17β per day, mean serum estradiol-17β concentrations were raised, respectively, 16, 32, and 67 pg/mL above baseline. At the same time, increases in estrone serum concentrations averaged 0.3, 9, and 27 pg/mL above baseline, respectively.[27]

It can be seen from Table 4 that estrone levels are much higher than estradiol levels in the postmenopausal woman treated with natural estrogens. If one considers estrone to have approximately 10 times less biologic activity than estradiol, then the 0.625 mg dose of conjugated estrogen, the 0.75 mg dose of estropipate, the 1.0 mg dose of micronized estradiol, and the transdermal estrogen patch releasing 50 μg/day of estradiol all approach the circulating estrogen levels seen in the early follicular phase of the cycle.

Progestin

An attempt has been made to compare the potencies of progestins used with natural estrogens or menopausal replacement therapy.[23] The dose – response relationship of the progestins on four different biochemical parameters in the endometrium and on the induction of secretory endometrial histology was examined and compared to results previously published in the literature. The consensus values for the dose of each progestin required to elicit secretory changes in estrogen-primed endometrium after six days of administration are shown in Table 5.

Table 5:
Oral doses of progestins required to elicit changes equivalent to secretory phase endometrium in estrogen-treated postmenopausal women

Progestin	Dose (mg)
Progesterone	200
Medroxyprogesterone acetate	5
Norethindrone	0.35
Levonorgestrel	0.075

Adapted from King R.J.B., M.I. Whitehead [23]

Conclusions

All of the natural estrogens, administered orally, result in equivalent serum estrone and estradiol levels and, therefore, there is no advantage of one over another. Parenteral, transvaginal, and transdermal delivery results in absorption of estrogen without rapid metabolism in the gut or by first pass effect in the liver. Natural estradiol is probably the estrogen of choice by these routes of administration. At the present time, it appears that any natural estrogen, delivered by any route, will have equivalent beneficial effects on estrogen sensitive target tissues and the choice of estrogen preparation should be a matter of patient and physician preference.

A progestin is typically added to estrogen replacement to prevent unopposed estrogen stimulation of the endometrium and endometrial hyperplasia. The lowest dose of progestin capable of inducing secretory endometrium, as outlined in Table 5, should presumably be used, since at these low-doses, it is likely that none of the available progestins has major adverse effects on estrogen mediated changes in lipid metabolism.

References

1. Bayard F., S. Damilano, P. Robel *et al.*, "Cytoplasmic and nuclear estradiol and progesterone receptors in human endometrium," *J. Clin. Endocrinol. Metab.* 1978, 46: 635-648.

2. Whitehead M.I., P.T. Townsend, J. Pryse-Davies *et al.*, "Effects of estrogens and progestins on the biochemistry and morphology of the postmenopausal endometrium," *N. Engl. J. Med.* 1981, 305: 1599-1605.

3. Leavitt W.W., W.C. Okulicz, J.A. McCracken *et al.*, "Rapid recovery of nuclear estrogen receptor and oxytocin receptor in the ovine uterus following progesterone withdrawal," *J. Steroid Biochem.* 1985, 22: 687-692.

4. Katzenellenbogen B.S., "Dynamics of steroid hormone receptor action," *Ann. Rev. Physiol.* 1980, 42: 17-36.

5. Welshons W.V., M.A. Lieberman, J. Gorski, "Nuclear localization of unoccupied oestrogen receptors," *Nature* 1984, 307: 747-749.

6. King W.J., G.L. Green, "Monoclonal antibodies localize oestrogen receptor in the nuclei of target cells," *Nature* 1984, 307: 745-747.

7. Wu C.H., T. Motohashi, H.A. Abdel-Rahman *et al.*, "Free and protein-bound plasma estradiol-17-β during the menstrual cycle," *J. Clin. Endocrinol. Metab.* 1976; 43: 436-445.

8. Neumannova M., A. Kauppila, S. Kivinen *et al.*, "Short-term effects of tamoxifen, medroxyprogesterone acetate, and their combination on receptor kinetics and l7β-hydroxysteroid dehydrogenase in human endometrium," *Obstet. Gynecol.* 1985, 66: 695-700.

9. Barlow J.J., C.H. Logan, "Estrogen secretion, biosynthesis and metabolism; their relationship to the menstrual cycle," *Steroids* 1966, 7: 309-320.

10. Fishman J., "Role of 2-hydroxyestrone in estrogen metabolism," *J. Clin. Endocrinol. Metab.* 1963, 23: 207-210.

11. Lin J.T., R.B. Billiar, B. Little, "Metabolic clearance rate of progesterone in the menstrual cycle," *J. Clin. Endocrinol. Metab.* 1972, 35: 879-886.

12. Ryan K.J., L.L. Engell, "The interconversion of estrone and estradiol by human tissue slices," *Endocrinol.* 1953, 52: 287-291.

13. Rigg L.A., B. Milanes, B. Villaneuva *et al.*, "Efficacy of intravaginal and intranasal administration of micronized estradiol-17-β," *J. Clin. Endocrinol. Metab.* 1977, 45: 1261-1264.

14. Casper R.F., S.S.C. Yen, "Rapid absorption of micronized estradiol 17-β following sublingual administration," *Obstet. Gynecol.* 1981, 57: 62-64.

15. Padwick M.L., J. Endacott, M.I. Whitehead, "Efficacy, acceptability and metabolic effects of transdermal estradiol in the management of postmenopausal women," *Am. J. Obstet. Gynecol.* 1985, 152: 1085-1091.

16. Anderson A.B.M., A. Sklovskye, L. Sayers *et al.*, "Comparison of serum oestrogen concentrations in post-menopausal women taking oestrone sulphate and oestradiol," *Br. Med. J.* 1978, i: 140-142.

17. Mashchak C.A., R.A. Lobo, R. Dozano-Takano *et al.*, "Comparison of pharmacodynamic properties of various estrogen formulations," *Am. J. Obstet. Gynecol.* 1982, 144: 511-518.

18. L'Hermite M., "Risks of estrogens and progestogens," *Maturitas* 1990, 12: 215-246.

19. Stanczyk F.Z., E.J. Mroszczak, U. Gocbelsmann *et al.*, "Plasma levels and pharmacokinetics of norethindrone and ethinylestradiol administered in solution and tablets to women," *Contraception* 1983, 28: 241-252.

20. Herbst A.L., "Diethylstilbestrol and other sex hormones during pregnancy," *Obstet. Gynecol.* 1983, 58(suppl): 35S-40S.

21. Sitruk-Ware R, B. deLignieres, P. Mauvais-Jarvis, "Progestogen treatment in post-menopausal women," *Maturitas* 1986, 8: 95-100.

22. Holzbauer M., "Physiological aspects of steroids with anaesthetic properties," *Med. Biol.* 1976, 54: 227-242.

23. King R.J.B., M.I. Whitehead, "Assessment of the potency of orally administered progestins in women," *Fertil. Steril.* 1986, 46: 1062-1066.

24. Hirvonen E, M. Malkonen, V. Manninen, "Effects of different progestogens on lipoproteins during postmenopausal replacement therapy," *N. Engl. J. Med.* 1981, 304: 560-563.

25. Kuttenn F., C. Rigaud, F. Wright *et al.*, "Treatment of hirsutism by oral cyproterone-acetate and percutaneous estradiol," *J. Clin. Endocrinol. Metab.* 1980, 51: 1107-1111.

26. Lobo R.A., P. Brenner, D.R. Mishell Jr, "Metabolic parameters and steroid levels in postmenopausal women receiving lower doses of natural estrogen replacement," *Obstet. Gynecol.* 1983, 62: 94-98.

27. Product Monograph for Estraderm®, Ciba-Geigy Canada Ltd., February 1992.

Treatment of Hot Flushes

Hot flushes are known to be manifestations of ovarian failure and subsequent estrogen deficiency. As such, hot flushes are most effectively treated by the replacement of a physiologic level of estrogen, which is the gold standard by which other therapies should be compared. It appears that estrogen doses necessary to stop hot flushes are generally higher than those needed to normalize calcium metabolism or to improve genitourinary atrophy.[1] Therefore, the rationale of titrating the estrogen replacement dose by elimination of hot flushes is a rational approach to the treatment of all menopausal estrogen deficiency conditions. The usual doses of estrogen needed to decrease hot flushes are 0.625 mg to 1.25 mg of conjugated equine estrogen or their equivalents in other estrogen preparations.

The association of hot flushes with waking episodes during sleep has been clearly demonstrated by polygraphic recording of the various stages of sleep.[2] It is not surprising, therefore, that Campbell and Whitehead[3] observed that women treated with estrogen replacement for severe hot flushes also had improvement of memory and decreased insomnia, irritability, and anxiety.

If estrogen replacement is contraindicated, other agents have been shown to decrease hot flushes significantly, although none is as effective as estrogen. The treatments include progestins such as medroxyprogesterone acetate, 10 to 20 mg per day;[4] clonidine, 0.1 to 0.2 mg per day;[5] and Bellergal-S, twice daily.[6]

References

1. Geola F.L., A.M. Frumar, I.V. Tataryn *et al.*, "Biological effects of various doses of conjugated equine estrogens in postmenopausal women," *J. Clin. Endocrinol. Metab.* 1980, 51: 620-625.

2. Erlik Y, I.V. Tataryn, D.R. Meldrum *et al.*, "Association of waking episodes with menopausal hot flushes," *JAMA* 1981, 245: 1741-1744.

3. Campbell S., M. Whitehead, "Estrogen therapy and the post-menopausal syndrome," *Clin. Obstet. Gynecol.* 1977, 4: 31-47.

4. Albrecht B.H., I. Schiff, D. Tulchinsky *et al.*, "Objective evidence that placebo and oral medroxyprogesterone acetate therapy diminish menopausal vasomotor flushes," *Am. J. Obstet. Gynecol.* 1981, 139: 631-635.

5. Edington R.F., J.P. Chagnon, W.M. Steinberg, "Clonidine (Dixarit) for menopausal flushing," *Can. Med. Assoc. J.* 1980, 123: 23-26.

6.   Lebherz T.B., L.T. French, "Nonhormonal treatment of the menopausal syndrome. A double-blind evaluation of an autonomic system stabilizer," *Obstet. Gynecol.* 1969, 33: 795-799.

Management of Genitourinary Problems

HRT has a most dramatic effect on complaints relating to changes in the lower genitourinary tract that is deprived of estrogen. Daily estrogen therapy for at least six weeks matures the urethral squamous epithelium.[1,2] It results in proliferation and improved vascularity of the epithelium, and usually fast relief of the symptoms of urgency, nocturia, and post-voidal dribbling. The effect on the vaginal mucosa is to increase thickness, and to decrease pH and vaginal dryness. General methods can be instituted either before or in association with hormone therapy, as advised in the section on Counselling (Chapter 5). Urethral dilatation will be necessary if narrowing of the urethra is impairing the free flow of urine.

Hormone therapy may be instituted with oral estrogen or vaginal creams, particularly if the main complaint relates to the genitourinary system. Oral or other systemic therapy for genitourinary symptoms usually requires a smaller dosage than that necessary for the treatment of vasomotor symptoms or the prevention of osteoporosis. Therefore, if the patient is on hormonal replacement for other postmenopausal complaints, the dosage will be adequate to treat or prevent symptoms arising from the lower genitourinary tract. Alternatively, daily treatment with 2 g ($\frac{1}{2}$ applicator) of conjugated estrogen vaginal cream (1.25 mg of conjugated estrogens) for two to three weeks will relieve the symptoms of vaginal atrophic changes or the urethral syndrome. The dose can be reduced to once or twice weekly as needed. It is important to realize that estrogen is rapidly absorbed from the vagina, and therefore results in systemic treatment. However, local therapy may be beneficial for a short time, along with oral estrogen, to promote rapid correction of genitourinary atrophy. There is no other effective treatment of atrophic vaginal changes. In patients with an intact uterus, the estrogen should be accompanied by a progestin.

References

1.   Smith P., "Age changes in the female urethra," *Br. J. Urol.* 1972, 44: 667-676.

2.   Walter S, H. Wolf, H. Barlebo *et al.*, "Urinary incontinence in post-menopausal women treated with estrogens," *Urol. Int.* 1978, 33: 135-143.

Management of Dermatological Problems

The skin of postmenopausal women tends to become dry, flaky, and thin. These changes are related to aging and estrogen deprivation but they can be reversed. Prospective studies have shown that skin collagen content can be improved in postmenopausal women by HRT.[1] However, optimum improvement depends upon closeness to menopause and the duration of treatment. The skin responds rapidly to estrogen therapy with or without a progestin. Skin collagen content and thickness can be restored if treatment is started early in the postmenopausal period and continued for about two years. After this time no further improvement occurs.[2,3] Skin thickness has been correlated with the metacarpal index (area of the cortex of a metacarpal bone) as a measure of the efficacy of treatment.[1]

Similar to the management of other changes that occur in the postmenopausal period, any hormonal therapy should be accompanied by general measures. Healthy skin reflects good nutrition in the form of a balanced diet and an adequate intake of essential vitamins and minerals. The dry, flaky condition should be treated with good (not necessarily expensive) moisturizers. Sunscreens should be used and exposure to sun should be limited.

References

1. Brincat M, E. Versi, C.F. Moniz *et al.*, "Skin collagen changes in postmenopausal women receiving different regimens of estrogen therapy," *Obstet. Gynecol.* 1987, 70: 123-127.

2. Punnonen R., "Effect of castration and peroral estrogen therapy on the skin," *Acta. Obstet. Gynecol. Scand.* 1973, suppl 21: 1-44.

3. Shahrad P, R. Marks, "A pharmacological effect of oestrone on human epidermis," *Br. J. Dermatol.* 1977, 97: 383-386.

Management of Psychological Issues

In the psychological evaluation of postmenopausal women, no significant difference is reported between those who were taking estrogen and those who were not,[1] though a positive relationship between symptoms of tension, anxiety, and irritability, and plasma estrogen levels has been reported. The studies that have been carried out have considerable methodological difficulties, not the least of which relate to sociocultural factors which are difficult to control.

Undoubtedly, estrogen therapy improves vasomotor instability and genitourinary symptoms. As a result, there is an improvement in sleep patterns, less fatigue, less irritability, and less interference with social activities. The evidence that estrogen has a direct effect on somatic complaints such as anxiety, headache, weakness, and fatigue is not so clear. The use of HRT is controversial, and has the potential to result in the treatment of a major affective disorder exacerbated by menopause in a totally inappropriate way.

The multiplicity of symptoms at menopause may create a diagnostic problem which can be resolved only by careful attention to the patient's presenting symptoms and the diagnostic criteria for depressive illness. A combination of short-term pharmacotherapy may improve sleep, libido, anxiety, irritability, and other subjective symptoms. Supportive psychotherapy, offered by the primary care physician or provided by referral to community-based counsellors, may serve to enhance self-esteem, inform the patient about the menopausal process, and validate the patient's concerns.

Reference

1. Coope J. "Double blind cross-over study of estrogen replacement therapy," S.J. Campbell (ed), *The Management of menopause and the Post-menopausal Years*, University Park Press, Baltimore, 1976: 159-168.

Management of Sexual Transitions

Hormone Replacement Therapy

HRT may have an indirect effect on sexuality. Vaginal dryness and associated mucosal changes, decreased sexual desire, and diminished response are among the sexual complaints of the postmenopausal woman. In those women who lack interest in sex as a result of these menopausal symptoms, an improvement in general well-being following HRT has led to a return of sexual desire.[1,2] However, progestins may diminish the favourable result obtained by estrogen alone.[3] A micronized preparation of progesterone, a 21-norsteroid progestin, is now available. It produces adequate plasma and tissue levels of progesterone. Further investigation is needed to determine whether it will antagonize the beneficial effects of estrogen and have less psychological side effects than the 19-norsteroid progestins.

Androgens are known to be potent stimulators of desire in initiatory behaviour, and are responsible for increased coital frequency and sexual satisfaction in both men and women although they have no direct effect upon vaginal lubrication, vasocongestive response, or orgasmic capacity. However, the addition of an androgen enhances sexual desire and is associated with increased orgasmic frequency and more sexual enjoyment.[4] Testosterone is not prescribed routinely, but only when lack of desire and diminished clitoral sensitivity do not respond to estrogen/progestin therapy. The average premenopausal woman makes about 7 mg of testosterone monthly. This decreases in the postmenopausal woman but remains substantial in women with intact ovaries. In patients with ovaries who are more than two years postmenopausal, there is a decrease in testosterone secretion to negligible levels. Often testosterone is administered in doses exceeding physiologic levels, with potential side effects of hirsutism, baldness, and deepening of the voice.[5] While estrogen deprivation and aging may not directly affect sexual activity, the use of androgens and estrogen/progestin therapy may be beneficial in initiating sexual activity after a period of abstinence or in patients who have had a total hysterectomy with bilateral salpingo-oophorectomy. With the availability of free serum testosterone determinations, one is able to maintain the free testosterone level within the normal range and limit the possible side effects.

Sex Counselling

Sociocultural attitudes and expectations play a significant role in the individual woman's interpretation and response to entering menopause. In contemporary developed societies, attitudes toward female sexuality and the place and meaning of sexual behaviour in a woman's life have changed in the last two decades.[6-9]

Menopause represents the beginning of a life phase that represents an average of 30 years, more than a third of a woman's lifespan. Women now hold expectations for a continuing and satisfying sex life.

When problems are encountered, therapeutic intervention will range from information, education, and reassurance to formal referral. The following schema[7] for evaluating and treating sexual disorders in menopause may prove helpful:

- elicit the sexual history and clarify its meaning and significance;
- assess the menopausal state and the effects of menopause-induced changes on sexual function;
- physical examination to diagnose menopausal changes and to detect pathological causes for sexual dysfunction;
- provision of information about sexual function in general and about changes that occur frequently at the time of menopause;
- initiate HRT when indicated;
- brief sex counselling, including specific behavioural suggestions by the primary care physician; and
- referral for further help to community resource personnel in the field of sex counselling.

References

1. Bachmann G.A., R. Lieblum, "Sexual expression in menopausal women," *Med. Asp. Hum. Sexual.* 1981, 15: 96b-96h.

2. Cutler W.B., C.R. Garcia, N. McCoy, "Perimenopausal sexuality," *Arch. Sex. Behav.* 1987, 16: 225-234.

3. Dennerstein L., Burrows G.D., Wood C. *et al.*, "Hormones and sexuality: effect of estrogen and progestogen," *Obstet. Gynecol.* 1980, 56: 316-322.

4. Sherwin B.B., M.M. Gelfand, W. Brender, "Androgen enhances sexual motivation in females: a prospective, crossover study of sex steroid administration in the surgical menopause," *Psychosom. Med.* 1985, 47: 339-351.

5. Rittmaster R.S., W. Wrixon, "Post-menopausal hormone replacement," *Nova Scotia Med. J.* 1990, 69: 83-86.

6. Bachmann G.A., S.R. Lieblum, E. Kemmann *et al.*, "Sexual expression and its determinants in the post-menopausal woman," *Maturitas* 1984, 6: 19-29.

7. Sarrel P.M., L. Sarrel, "Orgasmic difficulties: the role of the gynecologist," *Clin. Obstet. Gynecol.* 1978, 21: 191-203.

8. Hunter M., "Emotional well-being, sexual behaviour and hormone replacement therapy," *Maturitas* 1990, 12: 299-314.

9. Walling M.A., B. Anderson, S.R. Johnson, "Hormonal replacement therapy for postmenopausal women. A review of sexual outcomes and related gynecological effects," *Arch. Sex. Behav.* 1990, 19: 119-137.

Prevention of Osteoporosis

Epidemiology of Osteoporosis and Its Complications

Osteoporosis is a major health problem in Canada, causing fractures, disability, pain, and deformity in growing numbers of women. It frequently is the cause of a loss in height in older women. Since osteoporosis affects approximately one in four women after menopause, it is estimated that as many as 2.5 million Canadians may be at risk for occurrence of osteoporotic fractures during their lifetime. Epidemiologists expect that the number of hip fractures among older Canadians will climb from about 15 000 per year in 1988 to about 28 000 per year in the year 2021.[1]

It has been reported that osteoporosis accounts for 1.2 million fractures each year in the United States.[2] The American Arthritis Foundation blames osteoporosis for 700 000 fractures per year. More than 10 000 000 American women who have passed menopause are currently losing sufficient bone mass, and hence skeletal integrity, leading to osteoporosis.

Hip fractures cause more deaths, disability, and medical costs than all other osteoporotic fractures combined.[3] The rate of hip fractures is between 150 and 200 per 100 000 people aged 60 or over in the United States and Canada. By age 70, this rate may climb to 500 per 100,000.[1] The incidence of osteoporotic fractures is expected to increase progressively because of aging of the population.

In 1981, there were 11 102 hip fractures in Canada among people aged 65 or over, costing in excess of $100 million for acute rehabilitation and long-term care for that year.[1] A recent estimate of health care costs related to osteoporosis in the United States was over $6 billion per year.[4] The pressure on hospital facilities and personnel will continue to increase with the rising numbers of patients experiencing osteoporotic fractures.

Mortality

Hip fractures due to osteoporosis result in a mortality rate in the first year about 12% to 20% higher than in similar persons who have not had a fracture.[3] The extent of bone wasting throughout life, up to the critical event of a hip fracture, may determine survivability afterwards. A British study of 195 elderly women who sustained a femoral neck fracture after relatively minor trauma showed that 24% died within three months of the occurrence.[5] This study, presented at the 1987 International Symposium on Osteoporosis in Denmark, found that the bone mass of those who survived more than three months after fracture was significantly greater than the bone mass of those who died.

U.S. epidemiologists have linked survival to functional status before the fracture. Of those dependent upon others at the time of fracture, 30% to 65% died within a year. Skeletal integrity has considerable bearing on functional status and survivability.

In 1986, there were 1 023 deaths following femoral neck fractures in Canada, 369 males and 654 females. More than 90% of these deaths were of people 70 years of age or older.[6] Many of these fractures were associated with falls. Accidental falls were the 10th leading cause of death among women 65 years or older. They were the 15th leading cause of death among males of this age group.

Prevention of Osteoporosis

It is of paramount importance that every effort be made to prevent the development of osteoporosis in the menopausal population in view of the tremendous burden of morbidity and mortality which the disease imposes. Females should take an adequate amount of calcium throughout their childhood and early adult years. Attention should be given to those risk factors for the disease that can be avoided or minimized. It is important to consider giving estrogen replacement therapy in early menopause in order to reduce the relatively large bone loss that occurs at this time.

Hormone Replacement Therapy

There is clear evidence that estrogen replacement therapy decreases the rate of bone loss in menopausal women and protects against fractures of the spine,[7] hip and the forearm.[8-10] The mechanism by which estrogen protects against osteoporosis and fractures is not entirely clear, but is likely multifactorial. The detection of estrogen receptors on bone cells[11,12] suggests that there is a direct action of estrogen on the bone itself. Estrogen replacement also decreases sensitivity of the bone to parathormone, resulting in less mobilization of calcium from the skeleton. In addition, there is support in the literature for an effect to increase vitamin D synthesis and to increase directly calcium absorption from the gastrointestinal tract. Furthermore, estrogen may reduce the production of mononuclear cell cytokines, such as interleukin-1. These chemicals may act on the bone remodelling cycle to prevent increased osteoclastic activation and the resultant increased bone resorption, as discussed in the earlier section on Bone and Mineral Metabolism (Chapter 4). Estrogen, therefore, is known to slow down bone resorption.[13] Bone resorption and formation are coupled; a steady state is reached after a few months of estrogen replacement.

The addition of progestin to estrogen replacement may also result in a synergistic effect on bone to increase bone mass.[16-18] Both estrogen and progestin receptors have been demonstrated on osteoblasts[11,12] and it has been shown that estrogen stimulates progesterone receptors in these bone cells. Progesterone may therefore directly activate osteoblastic bone formation with the result being that the combination of estrogen and progestin replacement may actually increase bone mass.[14] Christiansen and Riis [15,16] have demonstrated that this is apparently the case in patients with documented osteoporosis. These investigators showed that a steady state is not reached for at least two years so that positive balance of bone formation versus resorption occurs for at least this length of time.

In order to retard bone loss in the postmenopause, most authors recommend a minimum daily dosage of 0.625 mg of conjugated estrogens or the equivalent. One study has suggested that a dosage of 0.3 mg of conjugated equine estrogen may be adequate in some women, provided that high-dose calcium supplements were taken.[17]

Other Possible Mechanisms

The ability of estrogen to protect against fractures may work through other mechanisms apart from an effect on bone mineral content. Estrogen may decrease the depth of osteoclastic resorption lacunae and therefore prevent trabecular perforation and disrupted architecture (disconnectedness). Another possibility is that estrogen may have an effect on bone matrix. This speculation is supported by work of Brincat *et al.*[18,19] who demonstrated that estrogen replacement therapy increases skin collagen content and that skin collagen and bone density appear to be correlated. It is possible that estrogen may increase collagen in bone matrix to make bone stronger and more flexible even though bone density is not increased.

This suggestion is supported by a study by Wallach and Henneman in 1959[20] in which the women were followed up for up to 30 years after menopause in the absence or presence of HRT. The women who did not receive HRT lost up to five inches in height as a result of vertebral compression fractures, whereas those women who were treated with estrogen within three to five years of the menopause had no loss in height for up to 20 years of therapy. Interestingly, when estrogen replacement therapy was started in women who had already lost height because of osteoporosis and vertebral compression fractures, the loss in height ceased, suggesting that estrogen was able to prevent compression fractures even though there was no obvious increase in bone density at this point. This study strongly suggests that estrogen has an effect on bone strength, likely acting through an effect on bone matrix to prevent fractures without necessarily altering the bone mineral content.

Finally, recent work by Crilly *et al.*[21] in London, Ontario suggests that estrogen may work through a third mechanism to prevent fractures by improving balance and by decreasing the incidence of falling. They demonstrated increased postural sway in menopausal women with Colles' fractures compared to control subjects and that this apparent decrease in ability to balance can be improved by estrogen replacement therapy.

Calcium Supplements

Evidence exists that during the period of growth and accumulation of bone, up to about the mid-thirties, an adequate intake of calcium is essential for the development of bone mass and to reduce the risk of subsequent fractures.[22] The daily amount of elemental calcium in the diet of North American women is between 475 and 630 mg.[23] Calcium metabolic balance studies have led to a recommended daily requirement of approximately 1000 mg of calcium before the onset of menopause and up to 1500 mg per day for postmenopausal women.[24] At the present time, it does not appear that calcium supplementation alone, even in massive doses, can prevent loss of bone mass in the presence of severe estrogen deficiency. However, it is clear that adequate calcium intake is required for HRT to be effective in protecting bone mass in menopausal women.

Calcium supplements are available in several forms (e.g., as chewable tablets, gelatin capsules, and effervescent preparations). The solubility of the most commonly used calcium salts – carbonates, and phosphates – is depressed as pH increases. Therefore, it is best to take these preparations with meals and with six to eight ounces of water or other fluids to enhance solubility. The solubility of other calcium salts, such as the citrate, lactate, and gluconate, are relatively unaffected by differences in pH.[25] Hypochlorhydria, common in the elderly, reduces calcium absorption, especially of the carbonate and phosphate salts.

Some Other Agents under Investigation

Fluoride

Despite the large body of evidence supporting a role of HRT on bone and mineral content, the actual mineralization of bone may not be the entire answer to protection against fractures. This premise is based upon studies examining fluoride effects on bone, as illustrated by the recent study of Riggs *et al.*[26]

They studied 202 postmenopausal women with osteoporosis who were randomized to receive either fluoride or placebo treatment together with calcium supplementation. These women were prospectively followed up for four years, during which time bone density and the number of fractures were monitored. In the fluoride group, bone density increased 35% in the lumbar spine and 12% in the femoral neck. In contrast, there was a 4% decrease in the bone density of the radial shaft, a predominantly cortical bone site. Despite the increase in bone density in the spine, there was no difference in fracture incidence between the fluoride-treated and the placebo-treated control group. However, there was a significant increase in nonvertebral fractures in the fluoride group compared to the placebo group. In particular, the fluoride group had a highly significant increase in incomplete or stress fractures of the lower extremity which may account for the very common side effect of lower extremity pain in patients on fluoride treatment.

To summarize, therefore, Riggs *et al.* concluded that fluoride treatment increased cancellous bone mass and slightly decreased cortical mass but resulted in increased skeletal fragility. There was no change in vertebral fractures and an increased incidence of fractures in cortical or cortical/cancellous sites in the fluoride-treated patients compared to control subjects. However, the use of lower doses of fluoride in other studies has suggested that fracture incidence is reduced. Therefore, fluoride therapy may be a potential treatment for osteoporosis but requires more study before a final verdict can be reached.

Vitamin D

Vitamin D is a steroid which is derived from sunlight and dietary intake. It facilitates calcium absorption from the bowel when calcium intake is low. Calcium absorption declines with age, both because of declining renal synthesis of 1,25-dihydroxy vitamin D_3 and because of declining numbers of vitamin D receptors in the small intestine. For both of these reasons, gastrointestinal calcium absorption declines and parathyroid hormone levels rise.

Secondary hyperparathyroidism thus produced is thought to be a major pathogenetic feature of age-related (type II) osteoporosis but this condition is often superimposed upon pre-existing postmenopausal (type I) osteoporosis. Moreover, there is strong evidence for a direct effect of 1,25-dihydroxy vitamin D_3 on bone cells. Vitamin D activates bone remodelling, stimulates differentiation of osteoclast precursors and directly stimulates osteoblast function.

A number of trials for treatment of osteoporosis with 1,25-dihydroxy vitamin D_3 have been carried out, including a recent large, controlled prospective trial demonstrating a substantial reduction both in spinal and long bone fractures.[27] Thus, while treatment with vitamin D remains investigational, it shows promise for the future.

Calcitonin

Salmon calcitonin (Calcimar®) is available in Canada for the treatment of Paget's disease and hypercalcemia. Some investigators consider it as an alternative bone anti-resorptive therapy in patients for whom estrogens are contraindicated. Calcitonin is a polypeptide synthesized in the thyroid gland and secreted in response to an acute increase in serum calcium. It appears to be a specific inhibitor of osteoclastic bone resorption.[28] The major disadvantages of calcitonin are its high cost, the development of biological resistance, and the need for parenteral administration. Intranasal use is being studied.

Diphosphonates

There is evidence that diphosphonates (also called bisphosphonates) may provide effective anti-resorption of bone through physical, chemical, and cellular mechanisms. Compounds such as etidronate (EHDP) (Didronel®) are available for use in Paget's disease and in hypercalcemia of malignancy. The diphosphonates are synthetic analogues of diphosphates, in which the oxygen atom linking the phosphates is replaced by a carbon atom, making the resulting compound resistant to biological degradation by phosphatase enzymes. Diphosphonates are "bone-seeking" compounds, to a variable extent, and appear to inhibit osteoclastic bone resorption.[28] Recent studies have suggested that these compounds may increase bone mineral content in postmenopausal women when given in a cyclical or interrupted fashion.[29,30]

A second generation diphosphonate, pamidronate (APD), was recently assessed in patients receiving long-term steroid therapy. After 12 months, the use of APD and calcium was associated with improved vertebral density and assumed a better pathological picture on biopsy compared with calcium alone.[31] Diphosphonates are still experimental and have not been indicated for the treatment of osteoporosis by either the Health Protection Branch in Canada or the United States Food and Drug Administration.

Summary

In conclusion, available data suggest that the combination of estrogen and progestin likely produces the greatest possible protection against osteoporosis and fractures in menopausal women. The mechanism of the protective effect is unclear, but may involve multiple actions such as change in the absorption of calcium from the gastrointestinal tract, a direct action on bone to decrease osteoclastic activity and to increase osteoblastic activity, an increase in the collagen and matrix of bone, and an improvement of balance which prevents falling. Other therapeutic agents have shown promise and are being tested as supplemental or alternative treatments.

References

1. Narod S., R.A. Spasoff, "Economic and social burden of osteoporosis," H.K. Uhthoff, E. Stahl (eds), *Current Concepts of Bone Fragility*, Springer-Verlag, Berlin, 1986: 391-401.

2. Riggs B.L., L.J. Melton III, "Involutional osteoporosis," *N. Engl. J. Med.* 1986, 314: 1676-1686.

3. Cummings S.R., J.L. Kelsey, M.C. Nevitt *et al.*, "Epidemiology of osteoporosis and osteoporotic fractures," *Epidemiol. Rev.* 1985, 7: 178-208.

4. Holbrook T.L., K. Grazier, J.L. Kelsey *et al.*, "*The Frequency of Occurrence, Impact and Cost of Selected Musculoskeletal Conditions in the United States*," American Academy of Orthopedic Surgeons, Chicago, 1984.

5. Aitken J.M., "Relationship between mortality after femoral neck fracture and osteoporosis," C. Christiansen, J.S. Johansen, B.J. Riss (eds), *Osteoporosis 1987. International Symposium on Osteoporosis, Denmark, 1987*, Osteopress, Köbenhavnk, Denmark, 1987: 45-48.

6. Kreiger N., "Osteoporosis in an aging population," *Chronic. Dis. Can.* 1988, 9: 85-87.

7. Lindsay R., D.M. Hart, C. Forrest, C. Baird, "Prevention of spinal osteoporosis in oophorectomized women," *Lancet* 1980, ii: 1151-1154.

8. Hutchinson T.A., S.M. Polansky, A. Feinstein, "Post-menopausal estrogens protect against fractures of hip and distal radius," *Lancet* 1979, ii: 705-709.

9. Paganini-Hill A., R.K. Ross, V.R. Gerkins *et al.*, "Menopausal estrogen therapy and hip fractures," *Ann. Int. Med.* 1981, 95: 28-31.

10. Weiss N.S., C.L. Ure, J.H. Ballard *et al.*, "Decreased risk of fractures of the hip and lower forearm with postmenopausal use of estrogen," *N. Engl. J. Med.* 1980; 303: 1195-1198.

11. Eriksen E.F., D.S. Colvard, N.J. Berg *et al.*, "Evidence of estrogen-receptors in normal human osteoblast-like cells," *Science* 1988, 241: 84-86.

12. Komm B.S., C.M. Terpenning, D.J. Benz *et al.*, "Estrogen binding, receptor mRNA, and biologic response in osteoblast-like osteosarcoma cells," *Science* 1988, 241: 81-84.

13. Snow G.R., C. Anderson, "The effects of 17-beta estradiol and progestagen on trabecular bone remodelling in oophorectomized dogs," *Calcif. Tissue Int.* 1986, 39: 198-205.

14. Prior J.C., "Progesterone as a bone-trophic hormone," *Endocr. Rev.* 1990, 11: 386-398.

15. Riis B.J., L. Nilas, C. Christiansen *et al.*, "Effect of oestrogen:progestagen treatment on bone turnover in early post-menopausal women," *Maturitas* 1984, 6: 169-170.

16. Christiansen C., L. Nilas, B.J. Riis *et al.*, "Uncoupling of bone formation and resorption by combined oestrogen and progestagen therapy in postmenopausal osteoporosis," *Lancet* 1985, ii: 800-801.

17. Ettinger B., H.K. Genant, C.E. Cann, "Postmenopausal bone loss is prevented by treatment with low-dosage estrogen with calcium," *Ann. Int. Med.* 1987, 106: 40-45.

18. Brincat M., C.F. Moniz, J.W.W. Studd *et al.*, "The long-term effects of menopause and of administration of sex hormones on skin collagen and skin thickness," *Br. J. Obstet. Gynaecol.* 1985, 92: 256-259.

19. Brincat M., C.F. Moniz, E. Versi *et al.*, "Decline in skin collagen content and metacarpal index after menopause and its prevention with sex hormone replacement," *Br. J. Obstet. Gynaecol.* 1987, 94: 126-129.

20. Wallach S., P.H. Henneman, "Prolonged estrogen therapy in postmenopausal women," *JAMA* 1959, 171: 1637-1642.

21. Crilly R.G., L. Delaquerriere Richardson, J.H. Roth *et al.*, "Postural stability and Colles' fracture," *Age and Ageing* 1987, 16: 133-138.

22. Matkovic V., K. Kostial, I. Simonovic *et al.*, "Bone status and fracture rates in two regions of Yugoslavia," *Am. J. Clin. Nutr.* 1979, 32: 540-549.

23. Heaney R.P., J.C. Gallagher, C.C. Johnston *et al.*, "Calcium nutrition and bone health in the elderly," *Am. J. Clin. Nutr.* 1982, 36: 986-1013.

24. Consensus Conference, "Osteoporosis," *JAMA* 1984, 252: 799-802.

25. Shangraw R.F., "Factors to consider in the selection of a calcium supplement," *Public Health Rep.* 1989, suppl 104: 46-50.

26. Riggs B.L., S.F. Hodgson, W.M. O'Fallon *et al.*, "Effect of fluoride treatment on the fracture rate in postmenopausal women with osteoporosis," *N. Engl. J. Med.* 1990, 322: 802-809.

27. Tilyard M.W., G.F.S. Spears, J. Thomson *et al.*, "Treatment of postmenopausal osteoporosis with Calcitriol or calcium," *N. Engl. J. Med.* 1992, 326: 357-362.

28. Lindsay R., "Alternative strategies for prevention of postmenopausal osteoporosis," *Public Health Rep.* 1989, suppl 104: 66-70.

29. Storm T., G. Thamsborg, T. Steiniche *et al.*, "Effect of intermittent cyclical etidronate therapy on bone mass and fracture rate in women with postmenopausal osteoporosis," *N. Engl. J. Med.* 1990, 322: 1265-1271.

30. Watts N.B., S.T. Harris, H.K. Genant *et al.*, "Intermittent cyclical etidronate treatment of postmenopausal osteoporosis," *N. Engl. J. Med.* 1990; 323: 73-79.

31. Reid I.R., A.R. King, C.J. Alexander *et al.*, "Prevention of steroid-induced osteoporosis with (3-amino-1-hydroxypropylidene)-1,1-bisphosphonate (APD)," *Lancet* 1988, i: 143-146.

Prevention of Cardiovascular Disease

Cardiovascular disease is the major cause of death in women in most industrialized nations. In women, the rate of death from cardiovascular disease increases dramatically after menopause. Although younger women have a much lower risk of dying from cardiovascular disease than men, this risk continues to rise with age, the incidence in postmenopausal women approaching that in men. There is now a significant body of evidence suggesting that estrogen replacement therapy in menopausal women is protective against the occurrence of heart attacks and strokes.[1-4] These data come from prospective cohort studies and retrospective case-control studies. In general, these studies demonstrate that cardiovascular disease mortality in estrogen replacement therapy users is between one-third and one-half that of nonusers (R.R.= 0.33-0.5). Estrogen replacement therapy also has been shown to be cardioprotective in women with pre-existing heart disease.[1]

Known risk factors for heart disease include age, smoking, hyperlipidemia, personal or family history of heart disease, vascular disease, or diabetes. The protective effect of estrogen replacement therapy is clearly observed even in women who are at high risk for cardiovascular disease.[2-4]

Cardioprotective Effect of Estrogen Replacement Therapy

Two cohort analytical studies have been published more recently. One study assessed both the mortality and hospital admission rates for myocardial infarction in a retirement community. For both study endpoints, postmenopausal estrogen use was protective.[5] The investigators also examined the rate of death due to stroke in the same populations. Again, estrogen use was protective.[6] A second group of investigators looked at the rate of cardiovascular death, from all causes, in American women recruited at 10 lipid clinics. The subjects, aged 40 to 69, were followed up for eight years, and again the estrogen users experienced a much lower cardiovascular death rate (R.R.=0.34), about one-third that of nonusers.[3]

These recent studies support the consensus view that estrogen replacement therapy protects against cardiovascular death, but it should be noted that they were non-experimental in nature. Since the addition of a progestin to the estrogen replacement regimen is rather recent, there is actually no information on the combined use of estrogen and progestin on the rate of cardiovascular disease.

To resolve the important issue of whether postmenopausal estrogen replacement is protective with respect to the development of cardiovascular disease, and the magnitude of this effect, a randomized trial is needed. Unlike the majority of the previously mentioned studies, it is important that a dose of a progestin be incorporated into the therapeutic regimens. Cyclical and continuous modalities of hormonal replacement need also to be evaluated. Accepting the scientific limitations outlined above, the majority of the studies supports a beneficial effect from estrogen replacement in the prevention of premature cerebrovascular and cardiovascular disease.

What is the mechanism of cardioprotection imparted by estrogen replacement therapy? In women, estrogen administered orally increases the level of high density lipoprotein (HDL) at all ages. In addition, it would appear that synthetic estrogens decrease the excretion and disposition of triglycerides, while increasing the synthesis of very low density lipoprotein (VLDL). The effect of postmenopausal estrogen replacement therapy is to lower concentrations of low density lipoprotein-cholesterol (LDL-C) and raise those for total HDL, HDL_2, and apoprotein A-I. The lowering of LDL-C was originally ascribed to estradiol valerate[7] and later confirmed for other preparations administered orally.[8-10] All of these changes are thought to have a protective effect in preventing cardiovascular disease. In general, women on estrogen replacement therapy have lower plasma cholesterol by 8 to 20 mg/dL (0.2 to 0.5 mmol/L) and lower LDL-C by 15 to 30 mg/dL (0.4 to 0.8 mmol/L) compared to age-matched control subjects. In addition, women receiving orally administered estrogen replacement therapy show a consistent 15% to 20% increase in HDL-C compared to control subjects.[11]

There are many alternative routes for the administration of estrogens, including transvaginal, transdermal and subcutaneous. The only study that looked at systemic effects of vaginally administered estrogens found no change in levels of HDL-C and LDL-C.[12] Short-term studies initially detected no significant effect of transdermal estrogens on lipoproteins.[10,13,14] A more recent study using percutaneous estradiol (estrogel) reported a significant decrease in LDL-C after 9 and 12 months of treatment, but no significant changes in HDL-C.[15] Two other more recent studies found only marginal changes in LDL-C and HDL-C after one to two years of using the transdermal route.[16,17]

The greater effect of oral administration of estrogen, as compared to the two other routes, is thought to be related to the higher concentrations of estrogen reaching the liver via the portal system, the so-called first-pass effect. Estrogen given via subcutaneous pellets or implants (presently not available in Canada) has been reported, in short-term studies, to elicit much greater responses of lipoproteins than those obtained with transdermal estrogen administration.[18,19] Reasons for these effects are not clear, but it is apparent that concentrations of estradiol absorbed from the subcutaneous pellet reach high levels in the portal circulation and have similar effects to those of orally administered estrogens.

Cholesterol Changes Related to Progestin Addition

A major recent interest is what effect the addition of a progestin to estrogen replacement therapy has on the cardioprotective property of estrogen. Although natural progesterone has no effect on either HDL-C or LDL-C concentrations, synthetic progestins (especially from 19-nortestosterone) tend to have opposite effects on HDL-C and triglycerides (TG) than estrogen. It appears that all available progestins for HRT antagonize the beneficial effects of estrogen on lipid metabolism, in a dose-dependent fashion. This adverse effect on lipids appears to be mediated through the androgenic activity of the progestins, resulting in an increase in plasma hepatic lipase activity which metabolizes HDL-C more rapidly.[20]

Cyclically administered conjugated equine estrogen (CEE, 0.625 mg/day), combined with medroxyprogesterone acetate (MPA, 5 or 10 mg/day for 10 days per cycle), has been reported to lower LDL-C by an average of 14% (range 12% to 18%).[17,21] There appears to be less consistency in the increase of HDL-C with combined CEE and MPA (mean increase 10%, range -6% to +25%). By contrast, postmenopausal women receiving mainly CEE have been reported to have 11% lower mean serum LDL-C, and 10% higher mean HDL-C than do untreated control subjects.[22-24]

Recent short-term (three to nine months) studies in small groups of women have evaluated regimens of continuous low-doses of estrogen and progestin.[23-27] Administration of 0.625 mg CEE daily combined with either 2.5 or 5 mg of MPA daily variably reduced serum LDL-C by an average of 14% (range +2% to -21%) and increased HDL-C by an average of 6% (range 3.5% to 12%). The effects of addition of a progestin when the estrogen is administered by the transdermal route are being evaluated.

Thus, recent data indicate that the lowering of LDL-C with HRT is preserved during the addition of MPA; however, definitive studies are required to ascertain whether MPA significantly alters HDL-C levels. Total monthly doses of 65 to 75 mg of MPA (cyclically or continuously) appear to have, at most, only small untoward effects on the beneficial lipoprotein changes (increased HDL and decreased LDL) induced by estrogen replacement therapy. More studies are needed to identify optimal regimens of estrogen and progestin replacement. However, it is likely that small changes in HDL or LDL may not be clinically relevant in view of the new data concerning the direct action of estrogen on the blood vessel wall (see below).

Relative Importance of Elevated Triglycerides

According to several authors, hypertriglyceridemia is not a coronary risk factor (see Gagné and Brun[28] for a review). Most epidemiological studies, however, do show a link between triglyceride levels and coronary artery disease (CAD).[29] Still, hypertriglyceridemia is associated with so many related phenomena, such as decreased HDL-C and obesity, that it does not stand out as an independent risk factor. These observations have, however, been mostly done in men. In women with low HDL-C and an LDL/HDL ratio greater than 3.5, it is known to be an important risk factor. Hypertriglyceridemia occurs more frequently than hypercholesterolemia, both in the general population and in patients with coronary disease.

Causes of hypertriglyceridemias are either genetic (primary) or secondary. Primary forms, such as hyperchylomicronemia and familial combined hyperlipidemia, are very rare. Secondary forms of hypertriglyceridemia are numerous and several are associated with CAD. Diabetes and obesity, often occurring together, are among the many pathologies associated with hypertriglyceridemia. There is a correlation between triglyceride levels and adiposity, particularly abdominal adiposity.

Estrogens, birth control pills, diuretics, beta-blockers without intrinsic sympathomimetic activity, and isotretinoin are often implicated in increasing triglyceride concentration. It is interesting to consider, however, that estrogen replacement administered by the transdermal route does not increase serum triglycerides.[13,14] Synthetic progestins tend to decrease circulating triglycerides.[15,16] This property is probably related to their relative androgenicity and to their effect on the metabolism of VLDL particles in the liver.

In the majority of cases, elevated triglycerides range from 2.5 to 6.0 mmol/L. In this instance, a family and/or personal history of CAD, the presence of other risk factors, diseases associated with CAD, low HDL-C, elevated LDL-C, and atherogenic tendency (high LDL/HDL ratio) are all elements that warrant consideration before administering HRT.

To assess the impact of progestins on cardiovascular disease, we must first examine the effects of combined estrogen/progestin therapy both on lipoprotein metabolism and on various other mechanisms whereby estrogens are thought to exert their beneficial actions. The effects of estrogen replacement therapy on insulin and glucose metabolism, coagulation and fibrinolysis, the prostaglandin/thromboxane system, and arterial blood flow all have been held to contribute to protection against CAD. Comprehensive studies to show whether progestins affect these areas are urgently needed. Although the precise role of triglycerides in the pathogenesis of CAD is controversial, it is likely that combined estrogen/progestin therapy will prove more beneficial than unopposed estrogen.[30]

Overall, we conclude that the use of combined estrogen/progestin therapy would not necessarily reduce the beneficial effect of estrogen replacement, if a suitable progestin is used; it would not negate the benefit of lowering LDL; and it may have a beneficial effect of lowering triglycerides. In any event, it would be wise to use the lowest dose of progestin necessary to protect the endometrium.

Evidence for Direct Effects of Estrogen on Blood Vessels

Recent evidence suggests that much of the cardioprotective effect of estrogen may be due to a direct action on the blood vessel wall. Estrogen receptors have been identified in the arterial walls of monkeys.[31] Estrogen appears to protect against atherogenesis by a direct action on the blood vessel wall to prevent or inhibit deposition of LDL-C.[32] Estrogen also appears to be able to prevent vasospasm, especially in atherosclerotic coronary arteries.[33] Estrogen may also act at the local level by increasing the production of prostacyclins by endothelial cells, thereby inhibiting platelet aggregation and atheromatous plaque formation. Prostacyclins may act directly to promote the vasodilatation associated with estrogen use.[34] This area is under intensive study.

References

1. Hammond C.B., F.R. Jelovsek, K.L. Lee *et al.*, "Effects of long-term estrogen replacement therapy," *Am. J. Obstet. Gynecol.* 1979, 133: 525-536.

2. Ross R.K., T.M. Mack, A. Paganini-Hill *et al.*, "Menopausal oestrogen therapy and protection from death from ischaemic heart disease," *Lancet* 1981: 858-860.

3. Stampfer M.J., W.C. Willet, G.A. Colditz *et al.*, "A prospective study of postmenopausal estrogen therapy and coronary artery disease," *N. Engl. J. Med.* 1985, 313: 1104-1049.

4. Henderson B.E., A. Paganini-Hill, R.K. Ross, "Estrogen replacement therapy and protection from acute myocardial infarction," *Am. J. Obstet. Gynecol.* 1988, 159: 312-317.

5. Paganini-Hill A., R.K. Ross, B.E. Henderson, "Postmenopausal oestrogen treatment and stroke: a prospective study," *Br. Med. J.* 1988, 297: 519-522.

6. Bush T.L., E. Barrett-Connor, L.D. Cowan *et al.*, "Cardiovascular mortality and noncontraceptive use of estrogen in women: results from the Lipid Research Clinics Program Follow-up Study," *Circulation* 1987, 75: 1102-1109.

7. Tikkanen M.J., E.A. Nikkila, E. Vartiainen, "Natural oestrogen as an effective treatment for type-II hyperlipoproteinaemia in postmenopausal women," *Lancet* 1978, ii: 490-491.

8. Knopp R.H., "The effects of postmenopausal estrogen therapy on the incidence of arteriosclerotic vascular disease," *Obstet. Gynecol.* 1988, 72(suppl): 23S-30S.

9. Barnes R.B., S. Roy, R.A. Lobo, "Comparison of lipid and androgen levels after conjugated estrogen or depomedroxyprogesterone acetate treatment in postmenopausal women," *Obstet. Gynecol.* 1985, 66: 216-219.

10. Fahraeus L., L. Wallentin, "High density lipoprotein subfractions during oral and cutaneous administration of 17β-estradiol to menopausal women," *J. Clin. Endocrinol. Metab.* 1983, 56: 797-801.

11. Wallace R.B., J. Hoover, E. Barrett-Connor *et al.*, "Altered plasma lipid and lipoprotein levels associated with oral contraceptive and estrogen use," *Lancet* 1979, ii: 111-115.

12. Mandel F.P., F.L. Geola, D.R. Meldrum *et al.*, "Biological effects of various doses of vaginally administered conjugated equine estrogens in postmenopausal women," *J. Clin. Endocrinol. Metab.* 1983, 57: 133-139.

13. De Lignieres B., A. Basdevant, G. Thomas *et al.*, "Biological effects of estradiol-17 in postmenopausal women: oral versus percutaneous administration," *J. Clin. Endocrinol. Metab.* 1986, 62: 536-541.

14. Chetkowski R.J., D.R. Meldrum, K.A. Steingold *et al.*, "Biologic effects of transdermal estradiol," *N. Engl. J. Med.* 1986, 314: 1615-1620.

15. Jensen J, B.J. Riis, V. Strøm *et al.*, "Long-term effects of percutaneous estrogens and oral progesterone on serum lipoproteins in postmenopausal women," *Am. J. Obstet. Gynecol.* 1987, 156: 66-71.

16. Stanczyk F.Z., D. Shoupe, V. Nunez *et al.*, "A randomized comparison of nonoral estradiol delivery in postmenopausal women," *Am. J. Obstet. Gynecol.* 1988, 159: 1540-1546.

17. Pang S.C., G.A. Greendale, M.I. Cedars *et al.*, "Long-term effects of transdermal estradiol with and without medroxyprogesterone acetate," *Fertil. Steril.* 1993, 59: 76-82.

18. Lobo R.A., C.M. March, U. Goebelsmann *et al.*, "Subdermal estradiol pellets following hysterectomy and oophorectomy. Effect upon serum estrone, estradiol, luteinizing hormone, follicle-stimulating hormone, corticosteroid binding, globulin binding capacity, testosterone-estradiol binding globulin-binding capacity, lipids, and hot flushes," *Am. J. Obstet. Gynecol.* 1980, 138: 714-719.

19. Farish E, C.D. Fletcher, D.M. Hart *et al.*, "The effects of hormone implants on serum lipoproteins and steroid hormones in bilaterally oophorectomised women," *Acta. Endocrinol.* 1984, 106: 116-120.

20. Tikkanen M.J., E.A. Nikkila, T. Kuusi *et al.*, "Reduction of plasma high-density lipoprotein-2 cholesterol and increase of postheparin plasma hepatic lipase activity during progestin treatment," *Clin. Chim. Acta.* 1981, 115: 63-71.

21. Miller V.T., R.A. Muesing, J.C. Larosa, "Lipid and lipoprotein changes due to estrogen replacement therapies and their association with prevention of cardiovascular disease in postmenopausal women," A.L. Goldstein (ed), *Biomedical Advances in Aging*, Plenum Publishing Corp., New York, 1990: 531-536.

22. Bush T.L., V.T. Miller, "Effects of pharmacologic agents used during menopause: impact on lipids and lipoproteins,"D.R. Mishell Jr (ed), *Menopause: Physiology and Pharmacology*, Year Book Medical Publishers, Chicago, 1987: 187-208.

23. Wahl P., C. Walden, R. Knopp *et al.*, Effect of estrogen/progestin potency on lipid/lipoprotein cholesterol," *N. Engl. J. Med.* 1983, 308: 862-867.

24. Rijpkema A.H.M., A.A. van der Sanden, A.H.C. Ruijs, "Effects of post-menopausal oestrogen-progestogen replacement therapy on serum lipids and lipoproteins: a review," *Maturitas* 1990, 12: 259-285.

25. Cano A., H. Fernandes, S. Serrano *et al.*, "Effect of continuous oestradiol-medroxy-progesterone administration on plasma lipids and lipoproteins," *Maturitas* 1991, 13: 35-42.

26. Moorjani S., A. Dupont, F. Labrie *et al.*, "Changes in plasma lipoprotein and apolipoprotein composition in relation to oral versus percutaneous administration of estrogen alone or in cyclic association with utrogestan in menopausal women," *J. Clin. Endocrinol. Metab.* 1991, 73: 373-379.

27. Yancey M.K., C.J. Hannan Jr, S.R. Plymate *et al.*, "Serum lipids and lipoproteins in continuous or cyclic medroxyprogesterone acetate treatment in postmenopausal women treated with conjugated estrogens," *Fertil. Steril.* 1990, 54: 778-782.

28. Gagné C., D. Brun, "Elevated triglycerides: how serious a risk factor? *Can. J. Cont. Med. Educ.* 1992, 4: 21-35.

29. Austin M.A., "Plasma triglyceride and coronary heart disease," *Arterioscl. Thromb.* 1991, 11: 2-14.

30. Crook D., J.C. Stevenson, "Progestogens, lipid metabolism and hormone replacement therapy," *Br. J. Obstet. Gynaecol.* 1991, 98: 749-750.

31. Adams M.R., J.R. Kaplan, D.R. Koritnik *et al.*, "Pregnancy-associated inhibition of coronary artery atherosclerosis in monkeys. Evidence of a relationship with endogenous estrogen," *Arterioscl.* 1987, 7: 378-384.

32. Wagner J.D., T.B. Clarkson, R.W. St. Clair *et al.*, "Estrogen and progesterone replacement therapy reduces low density lipoprotein accumulation in the coronary arteries of surgically postmenopausal cynomologus monkeys," *J. Clin. Invest.* 1991, 88: 1995-2002.

33. Williams J.K., M.R. Adams, H.S. Klopfenstein *et al.*, "Estrogen modulates responses of atherosclerotic coronary arteries," *Circulation* 1990, 81: 1680-1687.

34. Silferstolpe G., L. Enk, B. Kallfelt *et al.*, "Effects of exogenous oestrogens on the prostacyclin/thromboxane balance in oophorectomized women," *Maturitas* 1984, 6: 184-185.

6. Risks of Hormone Replacement Therapy

Neoplasia

Endometrium: Hyperplasia and Carcinoma

The incidence of endometrial adenocarcinoma rose sharply in the 1970s to become the most frequent malignant neoplasm of the female genital tract in North American women.[1] Stimulation of the endometrium by estrogen, unopposed by a progestin, is recognized as the major fundamental risk factor for hyperplasia and carcinoma of the endometrium. Hyperestrogenism can be either exogenous or endogenous. Whereas endogenous hyperestrogenism is associated with anovulatory cycles, estrogen-producing ovarian tumours, and obesity, exogenous hyperestrogenism is usually due to ingestion of estrogen for therapeutic purposes.

Unopposed estrogen, whether endogenous or exogenous, stimulates the endometrium to proliferate in a disorderly fashion and continued stimulation leads to endometrial hyperplasia. There is a morphologic continuum in endometrial hyperplasia ranging from mild (or cystic) hyperplasia through increasingly complex glandular (or adenomatous) patterns to the advanced stages with cytologic and architectural atypia. The latter may be so striking that even a pathologist may find it difficult to distinguish severe hyperplasia from well-differentiated adenocarcinoma. The risk of a hyperplasia progressing to a carcinoma depends upon the presence or absence of cytologic atypia in the epithelial cells. Only about 1.6% of patients with simple hyperplasia develop cancer as compared to 23% of those with atypical hyperplasia.[2] In uteri resected from patients with atypical hyperplasia diagnosed in curettings, 25% contained small superficial foci of well-differentiated adenocarcinoma.[3]

Epidemiological studies of several types have shown a positive relationship between the use of exogenous estrogens and the development of endometrial cancer.[4] These studies have included case-control and cohort studies as well as trend analyses correlating the incidence of endometrial cancer with prescriptions and sales of estrogens.

Most studies have suggested that the risk of endometrial cancer increases with increasing dose and duration of estrogen therapy. Current users of estrogens appear to be at greater risk than past users. As the increased risk is noticeable as soon as two years of use, it suggests that the role of estrogen is probably as a promoter rather than an initiator of carcinogenesis.

In the Cancer and Steroid Hormone Study,[5] women with unopposed estrogen replacement therapy for two to five years had a relative risk of endometrial carcinoma of 2.1, which increased to 3.5 for those with more than six years of therapy. The elevated risk persisted for more than six years. However, although the number of cases was small, those women who used conjugated equine estrogen preparations exclusively, at doses of ≤0.625 mg, had no increased risk of endometrial cancer. In a continuing large cohort study in a southern California retirement community,[6] the relative risk of endometrial cancer was 10 in estrogen users, increasing to 20 for over 15 years of therapy. Women who had last used estrogens more than 15 years previously still had an increased risk of 5.8. There was no dose-relationship in this study. It should be observed that the patients in these two studies had not taken a progestin in association with their estrogen replacement therapy.

Endometrial cancers in users of estrogen have a better prognosis than in nonusers.[7] Most cancers of the endometrium developing in women taking estrogens are well-differentiated Stage I lesions.[8] Myometrial invasion is present in only 30% and it is almost always superficial. Long-term use of high-dose estrogen preparations increases the risk of not only invasive endometrial carcinoma confined to the uterus but also for advanced lesions.[5,9]

Progestins can prevent the development of endometrial hyperplasia during estrogen therapy and can reverse established hyperplasia.[10] When estrogen is taken cyclically, the addition of a progestin has been shown to reduce the risk of endometrial hyperstimulation.[11] Long-term (five years) follow-up of patients taking 0.625 mg conjugated estrogens and cyclical 5 mg of medroxyprogesterone acetate (14 days per cycle) have shown no endometrial hyperstimulation (hyperplasia). In addition, approximately 70% of the patients have stopped bleeding.[12] Maximal beneficial effects are obtained when progestins are added for about 14 days during each calendar month whereas side effects are reduced by using the minimum dose of progestin.[13] As the addition of progestin might counteract the cardiovascular benefit of estrogen therapy, there is much interest in those potential advantages of newer progestins such as norgestimate, gestodene, and desogestrel.[14]

References

1. Weiss N.S., D.R. Szekely, D.F. Austin, "Increasing incidence of endometrial cancer in the United States," *N. Engl. J. Med.* 1976, 294: 1259-1262.

2. Kurman R.J., P.F. Kaminski, H.J. Norris, "The behavior of endometrial hyperplasia. A long-term study of 'untreated' hyperplasia in 170 patients," *Cancer* 1985, 56: 403-412.

3. Tavassoli F., F.T. Kraus, "Endometrial lesions in uteri resected for atypical endometrial hyperplasia," *Am. J. Clin. Pathol.* 1978, 70: 770-779.

4. Henderson, B.E., "The cancer question: an overview of recent epidemiologic and retrospective data," *Am. J. Obstet. Gynecol.* 1989, 161: 1859-1864.

5. Rubin G.L., H.B. Peterson, N.C. Lee *et al.*, "Estrogen replacement therapy and the risk of endometrial cancer: remaining controversies," *Am. J. Obstet. Gynecol.* 1990, 162: 148-154.

6. Paganini-Hill A., R.K. Ross, B.E. Henderson, "Endometrial cancer and patterns of use of oestrogen replacement therapy: a cohort study," *Br. J. Cancer* 1989; 59: 445-447.

7. Collins J., A. Donner, L.H. Allen *et al.*, "Oestrogen use and survival in endometrial cancer," *Lancet* 1980, ii: 961-964.

8. Silverberg S.G., D. Mullen, J.A. Faraci *et al.*, "Endometrial carcinoma: clinical-pathologic comparison of cases in postmenopausal women receiving and not receiving exogenous estrogens," *Cancer* 1980, 45: 3018-3026.

9. Shapiro S., J.P. Kelly, L. Rosenberg *et al.*, "Risk of localized and widespread endometrial cancer in relation to recent and discontinued use of conjugated estrogens," *N. Engl. J. Med.* 1985, 313: 969-972.

10. WHO, "Collaborative Study of Neoplasia and Steroid Contraceptives. Endometrial cancer and combined oral contraceptives," *Int. J. Epidemiol.* 1988, 17: 263-269.

11. Gelfand M.M., A. Ferenczy, "A prospective 1-year study of estrogen and progestin in postmenopausal women: effects on the endometrium," *Obstet. Gynecol.* 1989, 74: 398-402.

12. Gelfand M.M., "Recent advances in the management of the menopause," *Proceedings of the VIIIth World Congress on Human Reproduction Joint IVth World Conference on Fallopian Tube in Health and Disease*, Parthenon Publishing, New York, in press 1994.

13. Whitehead M.I., T.C. Hillard, D. Crook: The role and use of progestogens. *Obstet. Gynecol.* 1990; 75(suppl): 59S-76S.

14. Samsioe G., "Introduction to steroids in the menopause", *Am. J. Obstet. Gynecol.* 1992, 166: 1980-1985.

Breast: Carcinoma

About 10% of women in North America will develop breast cancer. The main risk factors for breast cancer[1] consist of:

- increasing age
- nulliparity
- late age at first birth
- early age at menarche
- late age at menopause
- personal history of benign breast disease or breast biopsy
- family history of cancer of the breast
- obesity in postmenopausal women

In women with a history of benign breast disease, there is an increased risk for carcinoma when atypical hyperplasia is present. The magnitude of the relative risk for these patients is 5.3 when compared to women with non-proliferative lesions on biopsy.[2] Women with atypical hyperplasia plus a positive family history of breast cancer were 11 times more likely to develop breast cancer than women without these findings.[2]

Recent evidence suggests that age at last birth may be an important factor.[3] Many other possible risk factors have been evaluated.[4] One cohort study failed to show that total fat intake or consumption of specific types of fat is positively associated with the risk of breast cancer.[5] However, a combined analysis of 12 case-control studies showed a positive relationship, particularly in postmenopausal women, for dietary fat.[6] Moderate alcohol consumption may contribute to an increased risk of breast cancer.[7,8]

Having important effects on the growth of breast epithelium, exogenous estrogens have been investigated as possible inducers or promoters of breast cancer. In a study comparing young Chinese women in the Far East and Boston, it was found that urinary estrone and estradiol were greatly increased in the high-risk Boston population in both follicular and luteal phase specimens as compared to the low-risk Far East population.[9] Increased levels of plasma estrogen have been found in postmenopausal women with breast cancer but information about body weight is not available. It seems likely that many of these women were obese with reduced levels of sex hormone binding globulin (SHBG) and increased free estradiol derived from peripheral conversion of androstenedione to estrone. However, increased levels of free estradiol and normal SHBG levels have been found in some non-obese women with breast cancer.[10]

The introduction of oral contraceptives was followed by concern about potential link of exogenous hormones with risk of breast cancer.[11] In the last 20 years, about 50 epidemiological studies have investigated this hypothesis. Recently, a few excellent critical epidemiological reviews of these studies have been published.[12-15] The authors separately tabulated results of case-control and cohort studies in relation to numerous different variables in order to calculate the relative risk for breast carcinoma in oral contraceptive (OC) users.[12-14] These studies were characterized by predominantly large population samples, different age groups, OC exposure, and were carried out in developed as well as developing countries. Several important conclusions can be derived from the analysis of this large body of epidemiological literature: there is a general agreement that most studies observed no increase in risk of breast cancer for women from developed countries who had ever used OCs, even with long duration of use or long time after exposure.[11,12] However, there are suggestions that oral contraceptives can increase risk of breast cancer for women in developing countries and for young women with benign breast lesions. This should be further investigated.[12] In addition, data derived from a few studies revealed a statistically significant increase in risk of breast cancer of premenopausal women exposed to long-term use of OCs.[12,13] The risk of breast cancer is not altered by different formulations of OCs.[11]

Several studies investigating the relationship between long-term non-contraceptive estrogens and the development of breast cancer have produced inconsistent results.[16-18] Moreover, adequate information is not available to assess differences among the various preparations of estrogens. A prospective study of nurses showed that current users who had been on hormone replacement therapy (HRT) for 10 to 15 years had an increased risk of breast carcinoma of the order of a third.[19]

Whereas the long-term use of high-dose estrogen replacement therapy may lead to a significantly increased risk of breast cancer, it is likely that short-term (less than five years) low-dose therapy using unopposed conjugated estrogens is safe.[20] The increased risk of long-term low-dose therapy is likely to be of the order of 30%[21] and should be considered in the context of other risks and benefits.

It is possible, indeed likely, that certain subgroups of women may be more susceptible to the carcinogenic effects of estrogens than others. Preliminary reports suggest that breast cancer risk following estrogen use may be enhanced in women with other risk factors for breast cancer.

Of further importance, in light of current medical practice, is the question of the effect of adding a progestin to estrogen replacement therapy. In the normal menstrual cycle, mitotic activity of breast epithelial cells is greatest late in the luteal phase when both progesterone and estrogen are present.[22] The theoretical concerns raised by this observation are obvious. Conflicting results have been reported on the effect of HRT with combined estrogen and progestin on the risk of developing carcinoma of the breast. One large study showed that progestin added to postmenopausal estrogen therapy significantly decreased the risk for breast cancer.[23] In contrast, a large population-based case-control study in Denmark reported that combined therapy possibly may be associated with an increased risk of breast cancer compared to treatment with estrogen alone.[24] Similarly, a Swedish study found a higher risk in women using combined therapy, but the number of patients in the particular subgroup was very small.[16] Therefore, we conclude that long-term HRT is associated with an increase in the risk of breast cancer, which might be increased by the addition of progestins.

The conflicting results of studies on this topic are particularly prone to various epidemiological biases in view of the lack of randomized clinical trials and the influence of known risk factors on prescribing practices, patterns of early diagnosis, and referral.[25] Nevertheless, the likelihood of a small increase in the risk of breast cancer should lead physicians to promote earlier detection, especially through screening mammography and the annual clinical examination of the breasts.

Increased surveillance may be particularly important for women on long-term HRT. There are now at least two papers in the literature which suggest that five-year survival is better for patients who develop breast cancer while taking estrogen replacement therapy than in age-matched controls who are not on HRT.[26,27] This suggests a situation analogous to endometrial cancer, in that breast cancer may be unmasked earlier by estrogen use and thus may be detected at an earlier stage prior to invasion.

The data presented in these epidemiological studies do not warrant a change in the current prescribing practice of HRT at this time, but the need for further investigation and ongoing surveillance must be emphasized. To ensure the lowest possible risk, however, it is reasonable to use the lowest dose of a natural estrogen which will stop hot flushes and protect against coronary heart disease and osteoporosis.

References

1.   Kelsey J.L., D.B. Fischer, T.R. Holford *et al*, "Exogenous estrogens and other factors in the epidemiology of breast cancer," *J. Natl. Cancer Inst.* 1981, 67: 327-333.

2. Dupont W.D., D.L. Page, "Risk factors for breast cancer in women with proliferative breast disease," *N. Engl. J. Med.* 1985; 312: 146-151.

3. Kalache A., A. Maguire, S.G. Thompson, "Age at last full-term pregnancy and risk of breast cancer," *Lancet* 1993, 341: 33-36.

4. UK National Case-control Study Group, "Oral contraceptive use and breast cancer risk in young women," *Lancet* 1989, i: 973-982.

5. Willett W.C., M.J. Stampfer, G.A. Colditz *et al*, "Dietary fat and the risk of breast cancer," *N. Engl. J. Med.* 1987, 316: 22-28.

6. Howe G.R., T. Hirohata, T.G. Hislop *et al*, "Dietary factors and risk of breast cancer: combined analysis of 12 case-control studies," *J. Natl. Cancer Inst.* 1990, 82: 561-569.

7. Schatzkin A., D.Y. Jones, R.N. Hoover *et al*, "Alcohol consumption and breast cancer in the epidemiologic follow-up study of the first National Health and Nutrition Examination Survey," *N. Engl. J. Med.* 1987, 316: 1169-1173.

8. Willett W.C., M.J. Stampfer, G.A. Colditz *et al*, "Moderate alcohol consumption and the risk of breast cancer," *N. Engl. J. Med.* 1987, 316: 1174-1180.

9. Trichopoulos D., S. Yen, J. Brown *et al*, "The effect of westernization on urine estrogens, frequency of ovulation, and breast cancer risk. A study of ethnic Chinese women in the Orient and the USA," *Cancer* 1984, 53: 187-192.

10. Siiteri P.K., G.L. Hammond, J.A. Nisker, "Increased availability of serum estrogens in breast cancer: a new hypothesis," In M.C. Pike, P.K. Siiteri, C.W. Welsch (eds), *Banbury Report 8, Hormones and Breast Cancer*, Cold Spring Harbor Laboratory, Cold Spring Harbor, New York, 1981: 87-106.

11. World Health Organization, "*Steroid Contraception and Risk of Neoplasia*," Technical Report Series 619, WHO, Geneva, 1978.

12. Thomas D.B., "Oral contraceptives and breast cancer: review of the epidemiologic literature," *Contracept.* 1991, 43: 597-642.

13. Khoo S.K., P. Chick, "Sex steroid hormones and breast cancer: Is there a link with oral contraceptives and hormone replacement therapy?" *Med. J. Austr.* 1992, 156: 124-132.

14. Stampfer M.I., G.A. Colditz, "The epidemiology of oral contraceptives and breast cancer," *Adv. Contracep.* 1990, 6(suppl): 27-34.

15. Romieu I., J.A. Berlin, G. Colditz, "Oral contraceptives and breast cancer. Review and meta-analysis," *Cancer* 1990, 66: 2253-2263.

16. Bergkvist L., H.-O. Adami, I. Persson *et al*, "The risk of breast cancer after estrogen and estrogen-progestin replacement," *N. Engl. J. Med.* 1989, 321: 293-297.

17. Brinton L.A., R. Hoover, J.F. Fraumeni Jr, "Menopausal estrogen and breast cancer risk: an expanded case-control study," *Br. J. Cancer* 1986, 54: 825-832.

18. Wingo P.A., P.M. Layde, N.C. Lee *et al*, "The risk of breast cancer in postmenopausal women who have used estrogen replacement therapy," *JAMA* 1987, 257: 209-215.

19. Colditz G.A., M.J. Stampfer, W.C. Willett *et al*, "Prospective study of estrogen replacement therapy and risk of breast cancer in postmenopausal women," *JAMA* 1990, 264: 2648-2653.

20. Palmer J.R., L. Rosenberg, E.A. Clarke *et al*, "Breast cancer risk after estrogen replacement therapy: results from the Toronto Breast Cancer Study," *Am. J. Epidemiol.* 1991, 134: 1386-1395.

21. Steinberg K.K., S.B. Thacker, S.J. Smith *et al*, "A meta-analysis of the effect of estrogen replacement therapy on the risk of breast cancer," *JAMA* 1991, 265: 1985-1990.

22. Anderson T.J., D.J.P. Ferguson, G.M. Raab, "Cell turnover in the 'resting' human breast," *Br. J. Cancer* 1982, 46: 376-382.

23. Gambrell R.D., R.C. Maier, B.I. Sanders, "Decreased incidence of breast cancer in postmenopausal estrogen-progestogen users," *Obstet. Gynecol.* 1983, 62: 435-448.

24. Ewertz M., "Influence of non-contraceptive exogenous and endogenous sex hormones on breast cancer risk in Denmark," *Int. J. Cancer* 1988, 42: 832-838.

25. Barrett-Connor E., "Postmenopausal estrogen and prevention bias," *Ann. Int. Med.* 1991, 115: 455-459.

26. Henderson B.E., A. Paganini-Hill, R.K. Ross, "Decreased mortality in users of estrogen replacement therapy," *Arch. Int. Med.* 1991, 151: 75-78.

27. Bergkvist L., H.O. Adami, I. Persson *et al*, "Prognosis after breast cancer diagnosis in women exposed to estrogen and estrogen-progestogen replacement therapy," *Am. J. Epidemiol.* 1989, 130: 221-228.

Ovary: Carcinoma

Despite a lesser incidence than endometrial carcinoma, ovarian carcinoma, with its much worse prognosis, is the leading cause of death due to malignancies of the female genital tract in North American women. The hypotheses that ovarian carcinoma might be due to high levels of pituitary gonadotropins and/or injury to the cells covering the surface of the ovary at ovulation result from the following two observations: (a) increased risk in those ovulating frequently (e.g., nulligravid women and treatment with fertility-enhancing drugs)[1] and (b) decreased risk in parous women and users of hormonal contraceptives.[2,3] Besides, other findings have incriminated environmental carcinogens, such as talc, and there is speculation on the role of estrogen and progesterone receptors that have been found in 52% of ovarian carcinomas.[4]

Earlier findings of an overall increased risk of ovarian cancer with stilbestrol[5] for menopausal therapy have not been replicated in other studies.[6] More specifically, estrogen use in menopause has been associated with both a protective effect for serous epithelial ovarian carcinoma[6] and a harmful effect for endometrioid ovarian carcinoma.[7] It is likely that the various histologic types of ovarian cancer have different etiological causes.

Investigation of the relationship between HRT and ovarian cancer is hampered by the lack of appropriate studies with extended duration of usage and adequate follow-up. In the absence of any good evidence regarding an association, the magnitude of any effect is likely to be small. Reliable information on the relationship will be obtained only through large epidemiological studies.

References

1. Whittemore A.S., R. Harris, J. Itnyre and the Collaborative Ovarian Cancer Group: Characteristics relating to ovarian cancer risk: collaborative analysis of 12 US case-control studies. II. Invasive epithelial ovarian cancers in white women. *Am. J. Epidemiol.* 1992, 136: 1184-1203.

2. The Cancer and Steroid Hormone Study of the Centers for Disease Control and the National Institute of Child Health and Human Development, "The reduction in risk of ovarian cancer associated with oral-contraceptive use," *N. Engl. J. Med.* 1987, 316: 650-655.

3. Depot-medroxyprogesterone acetate (DMPA) and cancer: memorandum from a WHO meeting. *Bull. World Health Organ.* 1986, 64: 375-382.

4. Kuhnel R., J.F.M. Delemarre, B.R. Rao *et al*, "Correlation of multiple steroid receptors with histological type and grade in human ovarian cancer," *Int. J. Gynecol. Pathol.* 1987, 6: 248-256.

5. Hoover R., L.A. Gray, J.F. Fraumeni, "Stilboestrol (diethylstilbestrol) and the risk of ovarian cancer," *Lancet* 1977, ii: 533-534.

6. Hartge P., R. Hoover, L. McGowan *et al*, "Menopause and ovarian cancer," *Am. J. Epidemiol.* 1988, 127: 990-998.

7. Weiss N.S., J.L. Lyon, S. Krishnamurthy *et al*, "Noncontraceptive estrogen use and the occurrence of ovarian cancer," *J. Natl. Cancer Inst.* 1982, 68: 95-98.

Vascular System Changes

Coagulation

Unlike the causal association between the oral contraceptive pill and venous thromboembolic disease,[1] there is no epidemiological evidence of such an association with HRT. This is likely to be due to the physiologic doses of natural estrogens used in HRT as compared to the higher doses of synthetic estrogens in oral contraceptives.[2]

There are two case-control studies that specifically address the question of whether estrogen replacement therapy predisposes to the development of venous thromboembolic disease. The first of these studies was part of the Boston Collaborative Drug Surveillance Program and compared the effect of estrogen replacement therapy to conventional oral contraception.[3] Unlike the positive association found in patients receiving estrogen in oral contraceptive doses, there was no increase in the rate of venous thromboembolic disease in women receiving estrogen replacement therapy. The selection of cases in this study excluded some women who were thought to have other risk factors for thrombosis. To clarify the situation, a second, more recent case-control study has been performed. In this study, 5.1% of the venous thrombosis cases versus 6.3% of the control subjects had received exogenous estrogen replacement, thus confirming that estrogen replacement therapy is not a risk factor for venous thromboembolic disease.[4]

Major epidemiological surveys of hemostatic variables and their association to ischemic heart disease indicate that increases in factor VIIc, factor VIIIc, and fibrinogen are all associated with both the presence and development of pre-mature ischemic heart disease. Of the above, factors VIIc and fibrinogen show the strongest correlation with ischemic heart disease.[5] Examination of postmenopausal women show that factors VIIc and fibrinogen are 6% and 10% higher, respectively, than in premenopausal women of the same age.[6] Some of the coagulation changes observed after menopause may be related to estrogen levels.

A double-blind crossover study of 22 women using conjugated equine estrogen showed a decrease in prothrombin time and a small increase in factor VII and factor X were demonstrated.[7] Another study compared the effect of conjugated equine estrogen 1.25 mg orally given daily for three weeks out of four for a period of three months, with estradiol valerate (2 mg), estrone sulphate (3 mg), and an oral contraceptive containing 100 µg of ethinyl estradiol and 2 mg of megestrol acetate.[8] This study showed no decrease in clottable factor anti-Xa activity (a measure of antithrombin III activity) for any of the medications except the oral contraceptive medication. Similarly, the prothrombin and kaolin cephalin times, plasminogen concentrations, platelet counts, and platelet function all remained unchanged except with the oral contraceptive medication.[9]

Experiments comparing the effects of transdermal estradiol and oral conjugated equine estrogens have examined the effects of these medications on fibrinopeptide A, high molecular weight fibrinogen, and antithrombin III (ATIII), measured both by functional and immunological assays. Fibrinopeptide A is a cleavage fragment produced during the conversion of fibrinogen to fibrin and is an exquisitely sensitive measure of thrombin generation. High molecular weight fibrinogen, an activation product of fibrinogen, has been shown to be raised in some patients on the contraceptive pill, and is thought to be a predictor of thrombosis. Transdermal estradiol in 24-hour doses of 0.025, 0.05, 0.1, or 0.2 mg and oral conjugated estrogens (Premarin) in daily doses of 0.625 or 1.25 mg did not alter hemostatic parameters to a degree increasing thrombotic risk.[10]

In summary, changes induced by currently prescribed doses of conjugated equine estrogens or small doses of natural estrogens, whether transdermally or orally, represent a completely different spectrum of response to the major effects observed with oral contraceptives. Specifically, the majority of studies examining levels of factor VIIc and fibrinogen during the administration of natural estrogens has not shown a clinically significant increase. The remainder of the above mentioned coagulation tests has not shown a strong correlation with premature atherosclerosis or an increased incidence of venous thromboembolic disease. Therefore, the studies that demonstrated small increases of various coagulation factors should not be interpreted as being primary evidence for an increased tendency to thrombosis.

It is recommended that estrogen replacement be accompanied by a progestin in women with an intact uterus. To date, no studies have demonstrated significant changes in the coagulation system due to short cyclical courses of progestins.

References

1. Special Advisory Committee on Reproductive Physiology, "*Oral Contraceptives 1994*," Health Protection Branch, Health Canada, Ottawa, 1994.

2. Lobo R.A., "Estrogen and the risk of coagulopathy," *Am. J. Med.* 1992, 92: 283-285.

3. Boston Collaborative Drug Surveillance Program, "Surgically confirmed gallbladder disease, venous thromboembolism, and breast tumors in relation to post-menopausal estrogen therapy," *N. Engl. J. Med.* 1974, 290, 15-19.

4. Devor M., E. Barrett-Connor, M.S. Renvall *et al*, "Estrogen replacement therapy and the risk of venous thrombosis," *Am. J. Med.* 1992, 92: 275-282.

5. Meade T.W., R. Chakrabarti, Y. Stirling *et al*, "Haemostatic function and cardiovascular death: early results of a prospective study," *Lancet* 1980, i: 1050-1054.

6. Meade T.W., A.P. Haines, J.D. Imeson *et al*, "Menopausal status and haemostatic variables," *Lancet* 1983, i: 22-24.

7. Poller L., J.M. Thomson, J. Coope, "Conjugated equine oestrogens and blood clotting: a follow-up report," *Br. Med. J.* 1977, 2: 935-936.

8. Thom M., M. Dubiel, V.V. Kakkar *et al*, "The effect of different regimens of oestrogens on the clotting and fibrinolytic system of the post-menopausal woman," *Frontiers Horm. Res.* 1978, 5: 192-202.

9. Meilahn E., L.H. Kuller, J.E. Kiss *et al*, "Coagulation parameters among pre- and postmenopausal women," *Am. J. Epidemiol.* 1988, 128: 908.

10. Chetkowski R.J., D.R. Meldrum, K.A. Steingold *et al*, "Biologic effects of transdermal estradiol," *N. Engl. J. Med.* 1986, 314: 1615-1620.

Hypertension

The majority of the studies on the effects of natural estrogens for hormonal replacement has either shown no change in blood pressure or a decrease in blood pressure.[1-3]

Two trials have specifically addressed the question of the effect of estrogen replacement on blood pressure. The first trial, performed in Britain, involved the randomization of 49 previously untreated postmenopausal women to placebo or one of six treatment groups comprising daily conjugated equine estrogen (1.25 mg), either with or without 5 mg of norethindrone acetate, piperazine estrone sulphate (1.5 mg) with or without the same dose of norethindrone acetate, and estradiol valerate (2 mg) with or without norgestrel (0.5 mg). Seventy-five percent of the patients experienced a fall in blood pressure compared to either pretreatment or the placebo group. This fall was small but was statistically significant.[4] A more sophisticated trial from Finland examined the effect of daily micronized estradiol (2 mg and 4 mg) in a randomized double-blind crossover study. This study examined the effect of this medication on both a normotensive and hypertensive group consisting of 10 subjects each. A significant fall in blood pressure was noted in each four-week cycle in both patient groups.[5]

In summary, there is no evidence that long-term estrogen replacement therapy predisposes to an increase in blood pressure. The majority of studies indicates that a slight decrease in blood pressure may occur. In the only study where a progestin was also examined, a decrease in blood pressure was also observed.[4]

References

1. Pfeffer R.I., "Estrogen use, hypertension and stroke in post-menopausal women," *J. Chron. Dis.* 1978, 31: 389-398.

2. Stern M.P., B.W. Brown, W.L. Haskell *et al*, "Cardiovascular risk and use of estrogens or estrogen-progestagen combinations: Stanford three-community study," *JAMA* 1976, 235: 811-815.

3. Barrett-Connor E., W.V. Brown, J. Turner *et al*, "Heart disease risk factors and hormone use in postmenopausal women," *JAMA* 1979, 241: 2167-2169.

4. Lind T., E.C. Cameron, W.M. Hunter *et al*, "A prospective controlled trial of six forms of hormone replacement therapy given to postmenopausal women," *Br. J. Obstet. Gynaecol.* 1979, 86(suppl 3): 1-29.

5. Luotola H., "Blood pressure and hemodynamics in postmenopausal women during estradiol-17β substitution," *Ann. Clin. Res.* 1983, 15(suppl 38): 9-121.

7. Guidelines for Hormone Replacement Therapy

In general, hormone replacement therapy (HRT) in a woman who has a uterus refers to the administration of estrogen in a dose sufficient to provide biological activity similar to that seen in the early follicular phase of a normally cycling premenopausal woman, and a progestin in a dose sufficient to prevent the development of endometrial hyperplasia.

Estrogen Regimens

The lowest dose of estrogen required to prevent menopausal flushes and to protect the bone against the development of osteoporosis should be used. This dose appears to be 0.625 mg of conjugated equine estrogen or its equivalent in other estrogen preparations as outlined in the section on Hormone Replacement Therapy: Pharmacology of Estrogen and Progestin Replacement (Chapter 5). Dose equivalents are approximately 0.625 mg conjugated equine estrogen, 1 mg micronized estradiol-17β, 0.75 mg estropipate, or 50 µg/day transdermal estradiol patch. If hot flushes are not relieved at this dose, then the dose may need to be increased up to a factor of two times.

Estrogen should be administered continuously, which may be particularly helpful for those patients who otherwise experience symptoms on the days off estrogen treatment. In a patient without a uterus, estrogen alone should be given continuously.

Problems Associated with Estrogen Use

If the patient has chronic active liver disease, or experiences gastrointestinal upset that persists with orally administered estrogen replacement, a switch to a transdermal estrogen delivery system should be considered. This method of delivery circumvents the first-pass effect of estrogen metabolism in the liver. A disadvantage is the possible occurrence of skin sensitivity reactions.

Progestin Regimens

In Canada, progestin is usually administered as medroxyprogesterone acetate, 5 to 10 mg orally daily, or norethindrone, 0.35 to 0.70 mg orally daily. Progestin is usually given cyclically. It appears that 12 to 14 days of administration of progestin are required to totally prevent the development of endometrial hyperplasia as a result of estrogen stimulation. In general, progestin is administered from the 1st to the 14th day of the month in patients receiving estrogen continuously. In those patients remaining on cyclic estrogen (1st to 25th day), the progestin should be given from the 12th to the 25th day of the month. Withdrawal bleeding may be expected to occur in up to 70% of patients in the days immediately following the withdrawal of progestin. Bleeding at other times during the month may be considered abnormal and should be investigated.

An alternative is to use a low-dose of progestin, such as 2.5 to 5 mg medroxyprogesterone acetate or 0.35 mg norethindrone, along with estrogen, continuously. This regimen of estrogen and progestin replacement appears to result in endometrial protection against hyperplasia or carcinoma while preventing withdrawal bleeding in the majority of women. The major drawback at present is the presence of irregular breakthrough bleeding, especially in the first few months of treatment, which may be confusing or worrisome to the patient or her physician. Other alternative forms of HRT are currently being developed and may be available in the near future.

Who Should Receive Hormone Replacement Therapy?

Perimenopausal Women (45 to 55 Years of Age)

Those women in the perimenopausal age group who develop chronic anovulation prior to complete cessation of ovarian function may experience periods that are irregular both in duration and in amount of flow. In these women, because estrogenic stimulation of the endometrium is not being antagonized by any endogenous progesterone production, the risk of endometrial hyperplasia or dysfunctional uterine bleeding is high. Endometrial sampling should be performed, and in the absence of hyperplasia, these women should receive cyclic progestin (i.e., 5 to 10 mg medroxyprogesterone acetate or the equivalent daily for the first 14 days of each month), in order to induce regular menstrual bleeding. This should prevent the occurrence of endometrial hyperplasia or carcinoma. Progestin administration alone, on a cyclic basis, should continue until such time as withdrawal bleeding ceases or the patient develops hot flushes, at which time estrogen replacement therapy also should be instituted. An alternative, in nonsmoking women, could be low-dose birth control pills.

Menopausal Women

In 75% of women, cessation of menses will be accompanied by hot flushes. The presence of hot flushes usually indicates estrogen deficiency. Estrogen and progestin replacement therapy as outlined above should be instituted.

In 25% of women, periods will cease but no hot flushes will be experienced. An evaluation of the endogenous estrogen status must be made to determine whether estrogen replacement therapy is necessary.

If the patient is thin, estrogen and progestin replacement usually should be instituted as described above. If the patient is obese, it is possible that she is making enough endogenous estrogen, from peripheral conversion of androgen to estrogen in fat tissue, to prevent the occurrence of hot flushes and to protect her bones against the development of osteoporosis. However, since this woman is at risk of developing endometrial hyperplasia from unopposed endogenous estrogen production, cyclic medroxyprogesterone acetate therapy is indicated to protect her uterus. Medroxyprogesterone acetate or another progestin should be administered for the first 14 days of each month as long as regular withdrawal bleeds occur. If the patient fails to withdraw following progestin treatment alone, estrogen replacement therapy should be added as outlined above.

In a patient without a uterus, hot flushes can be expected to occur around the age of 50. The hot flushes are indicative of estrogen deficiency; continuous estrogen replacement can be initiated. If the patient has not experienced hot flushes by the age of 50, a serum follicle stimulating hormone (FSH) determination should be made yearly. If FSH is low and indicative of continuing ovarian function, then estrogen replacement therapy is not recommended. Once serum FSH is seen to be elevated (over 40 IU/L), the patient is menopausal. If she is thin, estrogen replacement therapy is indicated. If the patient is obese and has an elevated FSH level, without hot flushes, it is likely necessary to obtain a serum estradiol level to determine estrogen status. If serum estradiol-17β concentration is under 50 pg/mL (150 pmol/L), then the patient should be started on estrogen replacement therapy.

Potential Contraindications to Estrogen Replacement Therapy

Breast Cancer

If the patient has breast cancer that has been treated, estrogen replacement therapy should be avoided. If the patient is experiencing hot flushes indicating estrogen deficiency, she is at risk for development of osteoporosis. A possible alternative to estrogen in this patient, to prevent distressing hot flushes and to protect against rapid loss of bone mass, is the use of progestin therapy alone on a continuous basis. Medroxyprogesterone acetate in a dose of 5 to 20 mg orally daily has been demonstrated to prevent or decrease hot flushes and to reduce calcium loss from the skeleton. Calcium supplementation in the range of 1500 mg/day is indicated in this patient.

Endometrial Cancer

For patients with Stage I, Grade I lesions treated with total abdominal hysterectomy and bilateral oophorectomy who have no or minimal myometrial invasion, estrogen may be used if the patient is estrogen deficient.

Patients with high-risk disease, namely patients with deep myometrial invasion greater than 50%, or positive peritoneal cytology or cervical involvement, or advanced stage disease, should not receive estrogen therapy.

Patients who are symptomatic who are not considered to be suitable candidates for estrogen replacement therapy can be treated with progestational agents for symptom control, such as medroxyprogesterone acetate.

Premenstrual-like Syndrome

If a patient has had moderate to severe premenstrual syndrome prior to the cessation of menses at menopause, she may experience a return of her depression, irritability, anger, and tension, as well as some physical symptoms such as breast tenderness and bloating, with the cyclic addition of progestin to estrogen replacement therapy for menopause. In such a situation, the patient may refuse any kind of HRT to avoid the return of her premenstrual syndrome symptoms. Because of the numerous benefits of estrogen replacement therapy and the very low risk of development of endometrial hyperplasia, such patients should be offered estrogen replacement alone with follow-up office endometrial biopsy once yearly or if intercurrent bleeding should arise to ensure that endometrial abnormalities are not developing. Combined (estrogen and progestin) continuous HRT also may be effective and would avoid the risk of endometrial hyperplasia or carcinoma.

8. Conclusion

Benefits and Risks of Hormone Replacement Therapy

Earlier sections of this report have discussed the manifestations, both major and minor, of the loss of ovarian function at menopause. The severity with which women experience symptoms of endogenous estrogen withdrawal, and the seriousness with which they perceive the changes that occur, is the result of education, communication among women, articles in the popular press and, to some extent, the cultural environment. Hot flushes and genitourinary atrophy produce symptoms that are disturbing, painful, and likely to encourage women to seek medical help. Associated conditions, such as depression, anxiety, emotional lability, sleep disturbance, and fatigue, interfere with the quality of life. The more serious manifestations of estrogen deprivation, such as osteoporosis and atherosclerosis, are more subtle, and may not trouble women until they have hip fractures or cardiovascular disease, when it is too late to prevent the problems.

Estrogen replacement therapy will alleviate all of the manifestations of endogenous estrogen withdrawal, with few side effects. The benefits are related to alleviation of vasomotor instability and urogenital atrophy, an improvement in the quality of the skin, and a delay in the onset of osteoporosis. There also is a reduction in cardiovascular and cerebrovascular morbidity and mortality. In recommending that women should consider hormonal replacement seriously, it is necessary to emphasize its preventive aspects, and to stress the need for compliant and continuing use.

The risks of hormone replacement therapy (HRT) are of major importance when long-term treatment is advocated. A concern is cancer of the endometrium resulting from the continuous administration of estrogen unopposed by a progestin. Progestins can prevent the development of endometrial hyperplasia and also reverse many established cases. When estrogen is taken, the addition of a progestin has been shown to reduce effectively the risk of endometrial hyperstimulation. It is suggested that women who have an intact uterus take a progestin together with estrogen in HRT.

The risk of breast cancer is a different problem. Breast cancer is a multifactorial disease which increases in frequency with advancing age. It is a common cancer in women. Several studies of the association of breast cancer with hormonal replacement have been conducted. Long-term estrogen use appears to be associated with about a 30% increase in the risk of breast cancer after a 10-year interval. Whether or not the concomitant use of a progestin increases risk is not yet completely clear. Nevertheless, it would seem inappropriate to deny women the other benefits of HRT because of a small increase in risk of breast cancer, providing women are informed of this risk and agree to accept it. It should be recommended, however, that monthly self-examination of the breasts be practised and an annual clinical examination of the breasts be performed. Screening mammography should be encouraged for women 50 years of age or older.

In contrast to the controversial situation with breast cancer, there are clear benefits in terms of increased life expectancy and quality of life due to decreased cardiovascular and cerebrovascular disease for postmenopausal estrogen users. These benefits, considered in conjunction with the positive effects on postmenopausal symptoms and the decreased incidence of osteoporosis, strongly favour the use of postmenopausal HRT.

9. Labelling

Guidelines for the Directions for Use of Oral, Transdermal, and Parenteral Drugs Containing Estrogen(s), at Low Dosages Appropriate for Hormone Replacement Therapy

(These form the basis of all advertising of estrogen-containing products for hormone replacement therapy to the medical profession from the pharmaceutical industry.)

and

Package Insert for Patients Using Estrogen Drug Products for Hormone Replacement Therapy

As Proposed by the Special Advisory Committee on Reproductive Physiology

Guidelines for the Directions for Use of Oral, Transdermal, and Parenteral Drugs Containing Estrogen(s), at Low Dosages Appropriate for Hormone Replacement Therapy

Clinical Pharmacology

To be supplied by the manufacturer.

Types of products in question are:

1. conjugated estrogens

2. esterified estrogens

3. estrogen as the single active component, natural or synthetic, or a combination of two or more estrogens

4. estrogen-progestin combination

5. estrogen-androgen combination

6. estrogen combined with other drugs

Indications and Clinical Use

Hormone replacement therapy (HRT) in cases of estrogen deficiency.

Contraindications

- known or suspected estrogen-dependent neoplasia except in special circumstances
- undiagnosed abnormal vaginal bleeding
- known or suspected pregnancy
- acute liver dysfunction or disease, especially of the obstructive type
- acute thrombophlebitis, thrombosis, or thromboembolic disorders

Warnings

- Before (drug) is administered, the patient should have a complete physical examination. Breasts should be examined together with mammography where indicated. Pelvic organs should be examined and a Papanicolaou smear should be taken.

- The first follow-up examination should be done within six months after initiation of treatment to assess medical response to treatment. Thereafter, examinations should be made once a year.

- If any surgical procedures are performed, the pathologist should be advised of the patient's therapy when specimens are sent for examination.

- If unexpected or abnormal vaginal bleeding occurs during therapy, diagnostic aspiration biopsy or curettage should be performed to rule out the possibility of uterine malignancy.

- Patients with acute hepatic disease, especially of the obstructive type, should not be given estrogens.

- Patients who develop visual disturbances, classical migraine, transient aphasia, paralysis, or loss of consciousness should discontinue medication. Acute disease is a contraindication but past history is not.

- If the patient develops any sign of phlebitis or thromboembolic complications, medication should be discontinued. Acute disease is a contraindication but past history is not.

Precautions

- Elevation of blood pressure in previously normotensive or hypertensive patients necessitates investigation but not cessation of medication because HRT has not been shown to increase blood pressure.

- Diabetic patients or those with a predisposition to diabetes should be observed closely to detect any alterations in lipid metabolism, especially triglycerides.

- When liver or endocrine function tests are indicated, or surgical procedures are performed, the laboratory should be advised of the patient's therapy before specimens are forwarded.

Adverse Reactions

List in order of organ systems involved and in order of frequency.

Symptoms and Treatment of Overdosage

To be described by the manufacturer.

Dosage and Administration

In women with an intact uterus, estrogen should be given continuously and with sufficient progestin to prevent overstimulation of the endometrial tissue. Unexpected or abnormal vaginal bleeding in such patients is an indication for prompt diagnostic measures. The lowest clinically effective dose of each hormone should be used.

Details to be supplied by the manufacturer on:

1.   Starting dose
2.   Maximal dose
3.   Usual maintenance dose
4.   Recommended duration of use

Availability of Dosage Forms

Description to be supplied by the manufacturer.

Package Insert for Patients Using
Estrogen Drug Products for Hormone Replacement Therapy

Estrogen Drugs

When a woman's menstrual periods cease (menopause) around the age of 50, the ovaries stop producing estrogens, the main female hormones. Sometimes the ovaries are removed by an operation causing "surgical menopause." Because estrogen deficiency is associated with a number of health risks, replacement of estrogens is recommended for the majority of menopausal women. In women with an intact uterus, estrogens are prescribed together with another female hormone called a progestin. This leaflet is designed to provide information about estrogen and estrogen/progestin therapy.

Uses of Estrogen

1. To Prevent Hot Flushes

When the amount of estrogen begins to decrease, some women develop very uncomfortable symptoms, such as feelings of warmth in the face, neck, and chest, or sudden intense episodes of heat and sweating ("hot flushes"). Hot flushes can cause frequent awakening at night, with sleep disturbance leading to fatigue, irritability, and depression. The use of estrogen replacement can stop or greatly reduce the occurrence of menopausal flushes.

2. To Prevent Osteoporosis (Brittle Bones)

After menopause, all women start to lose calcium from their bones at an accelerated rate. In time, this causes a thinning of the bones called osteoporosis which makes them weaker and more likely to break, often leading to fractures of the vertebrae, hip, and wrist bones. Taking estrogens after menopause slows down bone loss and may prevent bones from breaking. Eating foods that are high in calcium (such as milk products) or taking calcium supplements, weight-bearing exercises, and taking estrogens may also help prevent osteoporosis.

Those women who are likely to develop osteoporosis include those with a strong family history of osteoporosis or bone fractures in older ages, and those who are white, thin, smoke cigarettes, and do not exercise.

Women who have an early menopause or undergo removal of their ovaries at an early age are at greater risk of developing osteoporosis and at an earlier age.

3. To Prevent Cardiovascular Disease (Heart Attacks and Strokes)

After menopause, especially after surgical menopause, women may develop a pattern of lipid (fat) in the blood which may make the chance of a heart attack or stroke more likely. It appears that estrogen replacement therapy may change this lipid pattern back to a more protective, premenopausal type.

4. To Treat Atrophic Vaginitis and Urethritis

As a result of estrogen deficiency, changes occur in and around the vagina (causing itching, burning, dryness, painful intercourse) and urethra (causing difficulty or burning on urination, and frequent voiding). These changes may be reversed by estrogen therapy.

When Estrogens Should Not be Used

Since estrogens may stimulate the growth rate of certain cancers, you should not take estrogens if you have ever had cancer of the breast or endometrium (lining of the uterus). However, in certain situations, you and your doctor may decide that the benefits of the use of estrogen may outweigh the risks.

Dangers of Estrogens

Cancer of the uterus – The risk of cancer of the lining of the uterus (endometrium) increases the longer estrogens are used without progestin and when larger doses of estrogens are taken. Therefore, it is important to take the lowest dose of estrogen that will control your symptoms. The addition of a progestin to estrogen replacement appears to eliminate totally the risk of developing estrogen-related uterine cancer. In a majority of women, the cyclic use of a progestin may lead to the occurrence of regular menstrual bleeding which is to be expected.

There is a higher risk of cancer of the lining of the uterus if you are overweight, diabetic, or have high blood pressure. If you have had your uterus removed (total hysterectomy), there is no danger of developing cancer of the uterus. Consequently, the addition of a progestin to estrogen replacement therapy is not required.

Cancer of the breast – Some recent studies of the use of hormone replacement (estrogen with or without progestin) suggest an increased risk of breast cancer after long-term treatment. Other recent studies do not show this relationship. Adequate information is not available to assess differences among the various estrogens. The data presented in these epidemiological studies do not warrant a change in the current prescribing practice of HRT at this time, but the need for further investigation and ongoing surveillance must be emphasized.

Gallbladder disease – Women who use estrogens after menopause are slightly more likely to develop gallbladder disease than women who do not use estrogens.

Side Effects

In addition to the dangers of estrogens listed above, the following side effects have been reported with their use:
- nausea and vomiting
- breast tenderness or enlargement
- enlargement of benign tumours of the uterus (fibroids)

Monitoring Your Health While on
Hormone Replacement Therapy (HRT)

See your doctor regularly – While you are taking estrogen and progestin, it is important that you visit your doctor at least once a year for a physical examination. Regular breast examinations by a health professional as well as by self-examination are recommended. A mammogram (breast X-ray) is suggested every two years from the age of 50 onwards. If members of your family have had breast cancer or if you have ever had breast nodules or an abnormal mammogram, you may need to have more frequent breast examinations.

If you are taking estrogen without progestin, your doctor may take a sample of the lining of the uterus to make sure that it is normal. Any woman taking HRT who develops any irregular bleeding requires investigation.

Be alert for signs of trouble – Report these or any other unusual side effects to your doctor immediately:
- irregular or unexpected bleeding from the vagina
- breast lumps

Other Information

Good diet, weight-bearing exercises, and calcium supplements are important to help prevent osteoporosis. Check with your doctor.

Keep this and all drugs out of the reach of children.

How Supplied

Description of the particular product to be supplied by the manufacturer.